DIGITAL NURSING

Investigating the ways in which digital technology is transforming the roles of nurses and how they deliver care, this book explores how nurses can optimise patient care, enhance clinical decision-making, and improve healthcare outcomes in the information age.

The first half of the book emphasises the importance of nursing theory in guiding nursing practice and decision-making in the context of digital healthcare. Examining how technology is transforming their responsibilities and skillsets, it showcases the opportunities and challenges that nurses encounter in embracing digital tools to optimise patient care. Some of the thorniest challenges relate to ethical considerations, and an international selection of contributors discuss some of the key dilemmas and provide strategies for navigating the ethical dimensions of digital nursing. The second half of the book focuses on three case studies – using social media, wound care, and infection control. These chapters look at how digital technology is transforming specific aspects of nursing practice, providing concrete examples of the impact of technology on patient care and nursing efficiency. The book concludes with a discussion of emerging technologies and their potential implications for nursing practice, patient care, and healthcare delivery.

This text is a valuable resource for students, practitioners, and educators interested in how new technologies are integrated into nursing theory and practice, and the implications for person-centred humanistic care.

Matthew Wynn is a Senior Lecturer in adult nursing at Liverpool John Moore's University. His research interests include the digitalisation of nursing, the ethics of digital technologies in nursing, and clinical applications of digital technology in wound care and infection control.

DIGITAL NURSING

Shaping Practice and Identity
in the Age of Informatics

Edited by
Matthew Wynn

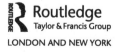

Routledge
Taylor & Francis Group

LONDON AND NEW YORK

Designed cover image: Image courtesy of Lisa Garwood-Cross

First published 2025
by Routledge
4 Park Square, Milton Park, Abingdon, Oxon OX14 4RN

and by Routledge
605 Third Avenue, New York, NY 10158

Routledge is an imprint of the Taylor & Francis Group, an informa business

British Library Cataloguing-in-Publication Data
A catalogue record for this book is available from the British Library

ISBN: 978-1-032-71451-6 (hbk)
ISBN: 978-1-032-71448-6 (pbk)
ISBN: 978-1-032-71454-7 (ebk)

DOI: 10.4324/9781032714547

Typeset in Times New Roman
by codeMantra

CONTENTS

     Louise Cave and Gillian Strudwick

     A vision for the future 141
     What is the future process of nursing? 143
     The start of the artificial intelligence (AI) revolution 144
     Clinical decision support 145
     Personalised care planning 146
     Health promotion 147
     Patient empowerment 148
     Robotics 149
     Remote monitoring 152

     Index   *159*

CONTRIBUTORS

Hannah Blake is Tissue Viability Clinical Nurse Specialist at Livewell Southwest. Her expertise includes tissue viability, lower limb management, pressure ulcer prevention, and digital technologies in wound care.

Louise Cave is Digital Operations Manager at The Hillingdon Hospitals NHS Foundation Trust and a Florence Nightingale Scholar. Her research focuses on digital, data, and AI in healthcare and nursing practice.

Mark Cole is Senior Lecturer at the University of Manchester. His expertise includes infection prevention and control, policy language, behaviour, and compliance.

Tiago Horta Reis Da Silva is Lecturer in Nursing Education at King's College London. His research focuses on nursing care for older adults, emotional intelligence, integrative medicine, and curriculum development.

Robert Douglas John Fraser is Adjunct Assistant Professor at Western University, London, Canada, and VP of Clinical Innovation at Swift Medical, Toronto. His research interests include wound care, digital health, big data, artificial intelligence, and analytics.

Lisa Garwood-Cross is University Fellow in Digital Health and Society. Her research focuses on health influencer culture.

Vanessa Heaslip is Professor of Nursing and Healthcare Equity at Salford University. Her research focuses on healthcare equity, social exclusion, and nursing leadership in digital healthcare.

Gillian Janes is Professor of Nursing and Quality Improvement at Anglia Ruskin University. Her research focuses on healthcare quality and safety, and nursing leadership in digital health policy and innovation.

Joshi Prabhu Navis is Lecturer in Adult Nursing at the University of Salford and interested in digital technology in nursing practice. Her past experiences include working as a clinical application analyst and a senior clinical research nurse using advanced therapeutic technology in diabetes care.

James Pearson-Jenkins is Senior Lecturer Education in Adult Nursing. Florence Nightingale Faculty of Nursing, Midwifery and Palliative Care, King's College London. His research focuses on pedagogy, especially on how nurse tutors develop resources in simulation and also propinquity in online group learning experiences.

Joanne Reid is Professor of Cancer and Palliative Care at Queen's University Belfast and a Global Nurse Consultant in Palliative Care. Her research focuses on patient involvement in palliative care and the use of digital technology in this population.

Louise Stayt is Senior Lecturer in Nursing at Oxford Brookes University. Her research interests include patient safety in critical care and digital solutions for post-critical illness rehabilitation.

Melanie Stephens is Associate Professor (Reader) in Adult Nursing at the University of Salford. Her research focuses on social care, interprofessional education, tissue viability, frugal innovation, and virtual wound care clinics.

Gillian Strudwick is Scientific Director at the Digital Innovation Hub and Chief Clinical Informatics Officer at the Centre for Addiction and Mental Health, Toronto. She is also an Associate Professor at the University of Toronto and specialises in digital health, mental health, and implementation science.

Cristina Vasilica is Reader in Digital Health at the University of Salford. Her research focuses on digital capabilities.

Marion Waite is Principal Lecturer at Oxford Brookes University. Her research explores technology adoption in healthcare, focusing on long-term health conditions and professional development.

Neil Withnell is Associate Dean at the University of Salford. His research focuses on digital capabilities and preparing the nursing workforce for the digital age.

PREFACE

Over the past few years, in countless conversations with undergraduate student nurses about digital technology, a recurring question surfaced: "Why is this relevant to us?" Many students, and indeed some practising nurses, asked this as they wrestled with the role of digital technology in nursing. "What does this have to do with our daily caring responsibilities?" These discussions revealed a significant hesitancy, sometimes even resistance, towards integrating technology into nursing practice. This reluctance isn't just limited to students. In fact, despite the obsolescence of fax machines, their use persisted in the UK until as late as 2022 (and likely beyond) within nursing services, requiring the health secretary at the time to formally ban their use. Meanwhile, in the US, nurses in San Francisco protested the use of AI in healthcare as recently as 2024 (Lydon, 2024). With one nurse reportedly claiming:

> We know there is nothing inevitable about AI's (artificial intelligence) advancement into healthcare. No patient should be a guinea pig, and no nurse should be replaced by a robot.

An Australian study (Wong et al., 2023) even highlighted a kind of professional identity crisis among undergraduate nurses as they confronted the reality of new digital tools; radically, calling on nurse educators to *prepare students to redefine their nursing identity*. While some regions, like Japan, have embraced robotic nursing, perhaps spurred by the realities of a super-aging society, elsewhere, a deep-seated fear remains that technology, for all its benefits, may dehumanise patient care.

These fears and questions are not just academic. The growing interest in nursing and robotics, underscored by a doubling of research articles indexed in PubMed between 2017 and 2023, reflects the urgency of understanding how our profession can and should evolve in response to digital advances. As I saw more of these concerns surface, it became clear that we need a new kind of conversation, a deeper exploration of what it means to be a nurse in a digital age.

This book was born from those conversations and from the pressing need to address the fundamental issues around nursing practice in this new era. But this is not a manual on how to use digital tools. Instead, it is a reflective exploration of what nursing is at its core, and how that identity might evolve alongside technological innovation. How do we maintain the essence of nursing while also embracing the incredible opportunities that digital tools present?

In a recent article, I suggested that nursing might not be a traditional profession with a clearly defined theoretical and epistemological base, as much as it is a social phenomenon (Wynn & Garwood-Cross, 2024). Unlike medicine, which typically focuses on the diagnosis and treatment of discrete pathologies, nursing is fluid. It is complex. Florence Nightingale herself recognised this when she wrote that a nurse's calling is diminished if they refuse tasks *because it is not her business*. In today's world, this insight is more relevant than ever. As nurses, we cannot afford to confine ourselves to old definitions or shy away from technology that may feel foreign. Our work touches every part of a patient's experience, and that now includes navigating virtual environments, artificial intelligence, and robotics, especially when these technologies affect clinical outcomes.

Indeed, we live in a time when digital technology's impact on well-being is indisputable. It's not uncommon to hear complaints about addiction to smartphones or the difficulty parents have in separating their children from digital devices. These tools have reshaped society, and by extension, they have reshaped nursing.

This book does not aim to prescribe rigid protocols for digital nursing; rather, it encourages deep introspection. It invites nurses to think about the sources of our professional identity, our intellectual authority, and how both must evolve as technology advances.

In the first chapter, we explore the essence of nursing through a sociological lens, asking, "What is nursing in a digital world?" From there, we move to the history of nursing theory and its applications in digital environments, including the rise of the "digital patient". In the second chapter, we examine how technology itself has influenced nursing practices using a socio-technical framework, drawing on insights from science and technology studies (STS). Subsequent chapters delve into the humanistic aspects of digital technology including inequalities, personhood, and person-centred care within the context of digital nursing, while also exploring the role of social media in innovating nursing practice and engaging patients. As one of my students once astutely remarked, *Our patients are online now; we need to meet them there.* The virtual environment has become as real and critical a space for care as the physical one, and it demands thoughtful engagement from all nurses.

The clinical chapters that follow provide concrete examples of digital innovations in infection control and wound care, both areas central to nursing practice. These case studies illustrate not only the successes but also the challenges of transitioning from non-digital to digital systems. In doing so, they highlight a question that has become essential to modern nursing: How do we balance new technologies with the deeply human aspects of care?

Infection control, for example, has long been a cornerstone of nursing. Florence Nightingale's pioneering work on sanitation and infection laid the groundwork for modern nursing, and today, infection control remains one of the most important areas of clinical focus. The recent COVID-19 pandemic, more than anything else, reminded us of this. The environmental impact on health, a key concern of Nightingale's, has now extended to a concern for *planetary* health, as highlighted by the Chief Nursing Officer's latest strategy for England. Wound care, another focus of the clinical chapters, represents perhaps one of the most enduring areas of nursing and medical inquiry, yet it too is undergoing transformation thanks to digital advancements.

In these chapters, we hear from both nurses and patients as they navigate this new landscape, providing a more tangible understanding of the real-world impact of digital nursing.

Finally, the book concludes with a vision for the future of nursing in the digital age. This is not just a call to action but a call to thought. We must actively shape our profession's future, ensuring that technology enhances patient care while preserving the human touch that lies at the heart of our work.

To summarise, this book is not a "how-to" guide. It is an invitation to reflect, to engage, and to embrace the complexities and opportunities that lie ahead. Digital technologies are changing the world at a rapid pace, and nursing is no exception. As we navigate these changes, let us remain rooted in the core values of our profession, ensuring that technology enriches, rather than diminishes, the humanity that is, and always will be, central to nursing.

References

Lydon, C. (2024, April). US nurses protest against the use of AI in hospitals. *Digital Health.* https://www.digitalhealth.net/2024/04/us-nurses-protest-against-the-use-of-ai-in-hospitals/

Wong, P., Brand, G., Dix, S., Choo, D., Foley, P., & Lokmic-Tomkins, Z. (2023). Pre-registration nursing students' perceptions of digital health technology on the future of nursing: A qualitative exploratory study. *Nurse Educator.* https://doi.org/10.1097/NNE.0000000000001591, December 25, 2023. | https://doi.org/10.1097/NNE.0000000000001591

Wynn, M., & Garwood-Cross, L. (2024). Reassembling nursing in the digital age: An actor-network theory perspective. *Nursing Inquiry*, e12655. https://doi.org/10.1111/nin.12655

ACKNOWLEDGEMENTS

As we present this book on digital technology and its profound influence on nursing professional identity and practices, I would like to extend my deepest gratitude to the remarkable group of co-authors who have contributed to this work. This book is the culmination of a truly collaborative effort, and it would not have been possible without the insights, expertise, and dedication of these distinguished nurses and scholars and the sacrifices they have made to invest time committing their thoughts and ideas to paper.

Each co-author brings a wealth of experience, representing the diverse fields of academia, clinical practice, and industry, including both nurses and experts from cultural studies and business IT backgrounds, making this an interdisciplinary project. Their collective experience spans multiple countries and continents, offering a global perspective on the challenges and opportunities that digital technology presents to the nursing profession. Their deep reflections on the implications of technology, coupled with their active engagement in its adoption and utilisation in practice, have enriched this book immeasurably.

Thank you for your unwavering commitment to this project and to the advancement of our profession.

Matthew Wynn – Editor

1

INTRODUCTION TO DIGITAL NURSING AND NURSING THEORY

Matthew Wynn, Tiago Horta Reis Da Silva and James Pearson-Jenkins

Introduction

This chapter explores the multifaceted nature of nursing, tracing its origins and formal establishment as a profession by Florence Nightingale in the 19th century. It delves into the challenges of defining nursing, reflecting on Florence Nightingale's broad yet ambiguous conception of the profession, and examines the evolution of nursing education and practice, emphasising the shift towards standardised training and professional registration. The chapter also discusses the impact of technological advancements on nursing, highlighting the potential risks and benefits of integrating digital technologies into practice. Through the lens of socio-political influences, it considers the changing roles of nurses, the quest for a distinct professional identity, and the importance of adapting nursing education to prepare for the challenges of the digital age. Finally, it provides an overview of the development of 'digital' nursing theory by contemporary theorists, and the advent of the 'digital patient'.

What is a nurse?

Understanding the impact of major technological advancement on a profession is challenging to achieve without first having a meaningful conception of what that profession is, what it does, and why it exists. The nursing profession arguably has its origins deep into pre-history given that the role of caring, a foundational focus of theories in nursing has always been necessary within human communities. Throughout most of history, these roles have typically been associated with women and class and historically had strong links to religious institutions. Typically, nurses learnt their profession via practice and experience rather than formal, standardised training regimes (Egenes, 2017). This changed in the 19th century with the reforms

DOI: 10.4324/9781032714547-1

to nursing and establishment of the first official school of nursing by Florence Nightingale at St Thomas's Hospital in London, within which a standardised curriculum was set and nurses learnt both in the classroom as well as at the bedside. This paved the way for the establishment of a professional register for nurses in 1921. However, these reforms to nursing education and legal requirements for registration to practise were not accompanied by significant efforts to define what nursing actually is. Indeed, the founder of the profession herself, Florence Nightingale was notably vague on this issue. Her philosophy on nursing is varied and included emphasis on the art of nursing and the importance of reflection on values and the concept of care; she was also pioneering in her use of statistics and evidence to inform her approaches to delivering nursing care. It is likely, as has been noted even in contemporary studies, that the existence and nature of the nursing profession have strong sociological features and was believed by Nightingale to be suitable for women due to their natural disposition for care work, which they already performed as wives and mothers (Gauci et al., 2023).

Critics have historically argued that efforts to regulate such a poorly defined profession have naively assumed that:

> ...all nurses would have the strength of character to assume a mature, professional approach to practise, as well as the ability to define their boundaries of their own performance within a professional and legislative framework designed to facilitate autonomy and creativity.
>
> *(Holliday & Parker, 1997, p. 487)*

This observation, if accurate, may account for the frequent observation that ritual plays a significant role in nursing practice. Rituals may bring a sense of structure and belonging to the profession. This feature of nursing practice is illustrated well in the context of wound care. A field currently (and uniquely) dominated by nurses in the UK (Guest et al., 2020). Studies undertaken throughout the last 20 years have consistently found ritualised and non-evidence-based practices to be prevalent within this area of care (Draper, 1985; Specht et al., 1995; Smith et al., 2010; Blackburn et al., 2019). This is despite major advances in the scientific evidence base in this field. However, in the face of rapidly developing digital technology these rituals are both threatened, and, in turn, threatening to the progression of a digitised paradigm of nursing. It is critical that new 'digital rituals' are not adopted. This is especially important given the impact of digital technologies to in some cases detach action from consequences or 'adiophirisation', a concept introduced by Bauman (1991). This issue was explored by Rubeis (2023) in the context of technology in nursing and considered that the reduction or 'dissembling' of the self into quantifiable parameters (as in the use of digital technologies for patient monitoring) has the effect of decontextualising vulnerability from individual experience. Rubeis (2023) provides some solutions to this issue in the form of calls to recognise the ontology of patients rather than simply seeing technology as a solution to a purely technical problem. However, ultimately this highlights the risks inherent in the development of digital technology use being ritualised in the same way traditional nursing practices have been performed. To understand these risks in more depth it is necessary to consider the factors influencing nursing practices in greater detail.

Nursing as a socio-political assemblage

To understand how nursing practices might, or should, change in the digital age, further exploration of what 'nursing' actually is must be undertaken. The identification and refinement of the 'metaparadigm' is an essential step in the ongoing evolution of the scholarly tradition in nursing. The nursing metaparadigm has long been considered to consist of four broad concepts which interact to govern the life-process, well-being, human behaviours, and the processes by which health is maintained. These concepts include the person, environment, health, and nursing (Fawcett, 1984; see Figure 1.1).

The 'person' considers the nature of individuals receiving nursing care. 'Environment' is the context of the human experience. Interactions with the environment may influence both health and the nature of the nursing process. 'Health' considers the dynamics between states of health and disease. Finally, 'nursing' is the academic and clinical practice of nursing professionals. It is important to note however that these four concepts were not defined clearly in the original scholarship on this theory. Contemporary nurse theorists have also noted that the metaparadigm in this

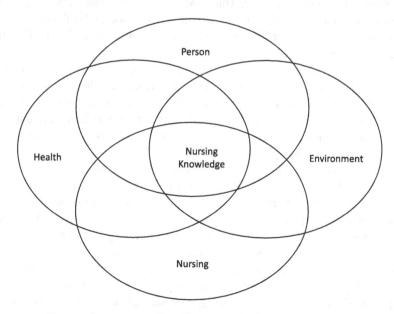

FIGURE 1.1   The nursing metaparadigm (Fawcett, 1984).

simplified form is unable to provide coherence which clearly separates nursing scholarship and practice from other groups such as doctors or allied health professionals (Bender, 2018). Another notable criticism of the nursing metaparadigm, to date the most well-known attempt to define the full scope of nursing practice, includes that one of the concepts is 'nursing'. Thereby requiring nursing practice to effectively define itself. However, this is viable if we consider that nursing practice itself is socially mediated and thereby a dynamic concept subject to external socio-political influences.

An example of the socio-political influences shaping nursing practice can be seen in the 2018 celebration by the Royal College of Nursing (RCN) of the first nurse in the UK to perform surgery independently of surgeons. This reflects a broader trend where nurses increasingly take on roles that were once the sole domain of doctors, likely driven by the growing complexity of healthcare services and demographic factors such as global ageing. That same year, the RCN also defined new standards for 'advanced practice' in nursing. While many nurses performing these roles do so with competence and contribute significant value to healthcare, there is a noticeable disparity in compensation compared to their medical counterparts.

This situation could be interpreted as aligning with what Paley (2002) refers to as a form of 'slave morality' in nursing. Originally a Nietzschean critique of Christianity, the concept of slave morality suggests that what are often seen as virtues, like 'turning the other cheek', are really mechanisms to manage behaviour. Paley adapted this critique to nursing, suggesting that nurses who acquire more skills are paradoxically seen as 'advanced' because they are willing to go 'above and beyond' in the name of care. This expectation, while noble, can obscure the fact that many nurses are taking on roles traditionally associated with higher-status and better-compensated medical professionals, without necessarily receiving the same level of recognition or reward.

This challenge in role definition has long been observed in nursing. Davies (1995) described nursing as essentially "the work which medicine rejects or fails to see" (p. 90). While there is nothing inherently wrong with nurses developing new skills that enrich their practice, it's important to recognise that these developments often reflect sociological forces rather than a coherent and independent definition of what constitutes 'nursing' itself.

Such considerations bring us to a Freirean challenge in nurse education. Freire and Ramos (1996) argued that critical education empowers individuals to recognise and challenge their oppression. In nursing, this could translate into awareness of the pressures to expand roles into medical and administrative tasks, often without corresponding benefits in salary or status. Addressing this dynamic through critical pedagogy might encourage nursing schools to move beyond the current competency-based approach, which assumes what nurses need to know, and allow for more autonomy in developing a critical professional outlook. Criticism of competency-based education is growing, with scholars like Collier-Sewell et al. (2023) calling attention to its limitations. Without recognising the broader social and political forces shaping their roles, nurses may struggle to develop a truly unique contribution to healthcare.

Some might ask why such a unique contribution is even necessary. This question can be countered by considering the value of a distinct intellectual framework for nursing – both as a safeguard against exploitation and as a way to predict how the profession might adapt in the face of transformative technologies in the digital age. However, it's worth noting that not all nursing scholars agree on the need for definitive theories to guide practice or on the necessity of defining nursing at all. Thorne (2023) argues that efforts to clearly delineate what nursing is are 'futile' and 'misguided', suggesting that theorising in nursing has largely been replaced by philosophising. While there is no clear evidence that nurses are more engaged in philosophy as a means of exploring practice, the reality remains: if nurses do not define their own profession, others, be they governments, healthcare administrators, or industry leaders, will do so on their behalf. These external definitions are shaped by many factors, including technological advances, the demands on healthcare systems, and broader social trends such as globalisation, litigation, and ageing.

Concerns about external influences on nursing identity are not new, and recent scholars have emphasised the importance of reversing this trend to protect nursing's identity as a distinct discipline. McCarthy and Jones (2019) offer valuable recommendations for how this risk may be mitigated.

1 It is essential to acknowledge that a lack of understanding of our nursing history may lead us to repeat past mistakes. Nursing education should incorporate an examination of how the field has evolved in today's society, taking into account the influences of structural and political forces, and ideology.
2 Curriculum development in nursing should be based on nurses' various forms of knowledge, preparing students for the intuitive aspects of practice that align with the discipline's ethical principles. Furthermore, students should grasp nursing as a narrative rooted in ethical principles and shaped by their ethical stance.
3 Beyond the introductory nursing theory course, it's important to establish mid-range and major theoretical perspectives as integral components of the curriculum, forming the basis for nursing practice throughout the entire educational programme.
4 We should encourage discussions in nursing education that consider the diverse perspectives and paradigms that influence nursing practice in our complex, postmodern world.
5 It's crucial to set examples and promote professional development that underscores the interpersonal aspects of nursing, recognising these as fundamental to nursing practice and acknowledging the personal challenges they entail.
6 We should advocate for a professional practice model that acknowledges the interconnectedness of personal and professional development. This model goes beyond the technical execution of medical regimens and places emphasis on understanding the full spectrum of human experiences.

These issues are critical in an age where digital technology is increasingly prevalent and has demonstrated benefits to both patients and nurses in addition to creating new sources of iatrogenic harm. According to Ziebland et al. (2021), the use of digital technologies can disrupt power relations leading to poorer clinical outcomes, 'e-iatrogenesis' (inadvertent harm caused to patients via the use or misuse of digital technologies), and create complex and potentially disruptive dynamics between professionals during the process of implementing new technologies. For nursing practice to adapt effectively to the demands and opportunities presented by digital technologies, it will be necessary for disruption of historic ritual as it manifests in nursing practice, and confusion as to the core purpose of nursing among nurses. It is challenging to argue for what should be a clearly definable scope of nursing practice, not least due to the seemingly limitless variation in roles nurses can, and do, undertake. The advent of highly networked and integrated digital systems, virtual care models, and the increasing use of the internet for clinical advice and information calls into question the moral and professional duties of nurses to act within these new digital environments.

Historical overview of nursing theory development

To better understand the direction of nursing and preserve its identity, it is necessary to examine the history and evolution of nursing theory as per the guidance of McCarthy and Jones (2019).

The evolution of nursing theory has been shaped by the contributions of visionary nurse theorists throughout history. From Florence Nightingale's pioneering work in nursing practice to modern theorists like Virginia Henderson and Paul Snelling, each has played a crucial role in advancing the profession of nursing. The following historical overview traces the development of nursing theory, highlighting key figures and their seminal contributions.

Florence Nightingale, who saw nurses as educated women in an era when women were neither employed in public service nor educated, is credited with founding the profession of nursing (Alligood, 2014a, 2014b, 2018). Modern nursing began with her vision and the founding of a school of nursing at St. Thomas' Hospital in London. Nursing has been acknowledged as an academic subject with a specialised body of knowledge as a result of the fast evolution of nursing theory over the past 60 years (Nightingale, 1859/1969; Bixler & Bixler, 1959; Kalisch & Kalisch, 2003; Fawcett, 2005; Alligood, 2010a, 2010b, 2014a, 2018; Alligood & Tomey, 2010; Chinn & Kramer, 2011; Walker & Avant, 2011; Im & Chang, 2012). Midway through the 1800s, Florence Nightingale sought to distinguish nursing knowledge from medical knowledge. According to her, a nurse's job is to prepare a patient so that nature may take care of them. Nursing theory was developed as a result of this (Nightingale, 1859/1969). As far as she was concerned, the correct role of a nurse was to best position the patient so that nature, or God, might work on him or her. She made the following point: unlike what doctors do in their profession, the knowledge that goes into caring for the sick is based on an understanding of the patient and their environment (Nightingale, 1859/1969).

Even with this early directive from Nightingale in the 1850s, the nursing community didn't start seriously discussing the necessity to build nursing knowledge apart from medical knowledge to guide nursing practice until 100 years later, in the 1950s (Alligood, 2014a, 2018). Prior to the 1950s, nursing practice was founded on customs and values that were passed down through hospital procedural manuals and the apprenticeship model of schooling (Alligood, 2014b, 2018).

The shift from vocation to profession involved several historical periods as nurses started to acquire a corpus of specialised knowledge to support their nursing practice. A major focus on practice was placed at the outset of nursing, and nurses strived to advance the profession over the course of the 20th century. From the standpoint of historical eras, progress towards the objective of creating a specialised foundation for nursing practice has been seen, acknowledging the push towards professional growth within each age (Alligood & Tomey, 1997; Alligood, 2010a, 2014a, 2014b, 2018). The curriculum era attempted to develop a standardised curriculum by addressing the issue of what subjects nurses should acquire to become qualified as nurses. A standardised curriculum was developed in the middle of the 1930s and was used by several diploma programmes (Alligood, 2010a, 2018). Nevertheless, many governments did not take action towards this aim until the middle of the 20th century, and in the latter part of the century, diploma programmes started to close while a sizable number of nursing education programmes were established in colleges and universities (Alligood, 2014a, 2018). Indeed, many countries to this day do not have standard training processes or even regulation of nursing professionals.

The trend of nurses pursuing higher education degrees gave rise to the age of research concentration. As more nurse leaders accepted higher education and came to a shared knowledge of the scientific age, this period was underway by the middle of the 20th century. Research modules were included in the nursing curriculum of early growing graduate nursing programmes, and nurses started taking part in research (Fawcett, 1978; Nicoll, 1986; Alligood, 2010a, 2014a, 2018). In response to the public requirement for nurses with specialised clinical nursing practice, master's degree programmes were developed as the research and graduate education eras evolved simultaneously. Nursing began to receive recognition and acceptability as an academic field in higher education, with the bachelor's degree gaining widespread acceptance as the first educational level for professional nursing (Meleis, 2007; Alligood, 2010a, 2014b, 2018).

The theory era in nursing has been a natural outgrowth of the research and graduate education eras (Alligood, 2010a, 2014a, 2014b, 2018; Im & Chang, 2012). The proliferation of nursing doctoral programmes from the 1970s and nursing theory literature substantiated the need for academic nurses (Nicoll, 1986, 1992, 1997; Reed et al., 2003; Reed & Shearer, 2009, 2012; Alligood, 2014a, 2018). As understanding of research and knowledge development increased, it became evident that research without conceptual and theoretical frameworks produced isolated information (Hardy, 1974; Batey, 1977; Fawcett, 1978; Alligood, 2014a, 2014b, 2018). Doctoral education in nursing began to flourish with the introduction of new programmes and a strong emphasis on theory development and testing (Fitzpatrick & Whall, 1983; Fawcett, 1984; Alligood, 2014a).

The 1980s was a period of major developments in nursing theory, transitioning from the pre-paradigm to the paradigm period (Kuhn, 1970; Hardy, 1974; Fawcett, 1984; Alligood, 2014a, 2018). Fawcett's proposal of four global nursing concepts as a nursing metaparadigm served as an organising structure for existing nursing frameworks and introduced a way of organising individual theoretical works in a meaningful structure (Fawcett, 1978, 1984, 1993; Fitzpatrick & Whall, 1983; Alligood, 2014a, 2014b, 2018). Classifying nursing models as paradigms within a metaparadigm of the person, environment, health, and nursing concepts systematically united the nursing theoretical works for the discipline, clarifying and improving comprehension of knowledge development by positioning theorists' works in a larger context (Fawcett, 2005; Alligood, 2018). The body of nursing science and research, education, administration, and practice continue to expand through nursing scholarship. In the last decades of the 20th century, emphasis shifted from learning about the theorists to utilisation of the theoretical works to generate research questions, guide practice, and organise curricula (Alligood, 2014a, 2014b, 2018). Evidence of this growth of theoretical works has proliferated in presentations at national and international conferences, newsletters, journals, and books written by nurse scientists who are members of societies as communities of scholars for nursing models and theories (Alligood, 2004, 2014a, 2014b, 2018; Parker, 2006; Fawcett & Garity, 2009; Im & Chang, 2012).

The theory utilisation era has restored a balance between research and practice for knowledge development in the discipline of nursing. New theories and methodologies from qualitative research approaches continue to expand ways of knowing among nurse scientists (Nicoll, 1986, 1992, 1997; Reed et al., 2003; Alligood, 2010a, 2010b, 2014a, 2014b, 2018; Wood, 2010; Reed & Shearer, 2012). The utilisation of nursing models, theories, and middle-range theories for the thought and action of nursing practice contributes important evidence for quality care in all areas of practice in the 21st century (Fawcett, 2005; Peterson, 2008; Smith & Leihr, 2008; Fawcett & Garity, 2009; Alligood, 2010b, 2014a, 2014b, 2018; Wood, 2010). An overview of this process in its entirety can be seen in Table 1.1.

The contributions of some key nursing scholars during the period of nursing progression to an established profession are provided:

Florence Nightingale (b.1820, d.1910):

Florence Nightingale, often hailed as the founder of modern nursing, revolutionised healthcare by introducing systematic practices and evidence-based approaches to nursing care. Her seminal work, "Notes on Nursing", published in 1859, emphasised the importance of sanitation, hygiene, and environmental factors in promoting patient health and recovery. Nightingale's holistic approach to nursing laid the

TABLE 1.1 Historical eras of nursing's search for knowledge

Historical Eras	Years	Major Questions	Emphasis	Outcomes	Emerging Goal
Curriculum Era	1900–1940	What curriculum content should student nurses study to be nurses?	Courses included in nursing programmes	Standardised curricula for diploma programmes	Develop specialised knowledge and higher education
Research Era:	1950–1970s	What is the focus for nursing research?	Role of nurses and what to research	Problem studies and studies of nurses	Isolated studies do not yield unified knowledge
Graduate Education Era	1950–1970s	What knowledge is needed for the practice of nursing?	Carving out an advanced role and basis for nursing practice	Nurses have an important role in health care	Focus graduate education on knowledge development
Theory Era:	1980–1990s	How do these frameworks guide research and practice?	There are many ways to think about nursing	Nursing theoretical works shift the focus to the patient	Theories guide nursing research and practice
Theory Utilisation Era:	Twenty-first century	What new theories are needed to produce evidence of quality care?	Nursing theory guides research, practice, education, and administration	Middle-range theory may be from quantitative or qualitative approaches	Nursing frameworks produce knowledge (evidence) for quality care

Source: Alligood (2014a, 2018).

foundation for modern nursing theory and practice, emphasising the nurse's role in facilitating healing and promoting well-being (Alligood, 2014a, 2018).

Mary Seacole (b.1805, d.1881):

Mary Seacole, a Jamaican nurse and contemporary of Florence Nightingale, made significant contributions to nursing during the Crimean War. Despite facing racial and gender discrimination, Seacole established the "British Hotel" near the battlefront, providing care and support to wounded soldiers. Her memoir, "Wonderful Adventures of Mrs. Seacole in Many Lands", documented her experiences and highlighted the importance of cultural competence, compassion, and resilience in nursing practice.

Clara Barton (b.1821, d.1912):

Clara Barton, known as the "Angel of the Battlefield", was a pioneering nurse and humanitarian. She played a pivotal role in establishing the American Red Cross and providing medical care to soldiers during the American Civil War. Barton's dedication to humanitarian aid and disaster relief laid the groundwork for modern emergency nursing and public health initiatives.

Dorothea Dix (b.1802, d.1887):

Dorothea Dix was a pioneering nurse, social reformer, and advocate for mental health care reform. She played a key role in establishing mental health institutions and advocating for humane treatment for individuals with mental illness. Dix's advocacy efforts led to significant reforms in mental health policy and laid the groundwork for modern psychiatric nursing.

Hildegard E. Peplau (b.1909, d.1999): Theory of Interpersonal Relations

Known as the "mother of psychiatric nursing", Hildegard E. Peplau is a well-known author, educator, clinical and theoretical specialist, and nursing leader. As the American Nurses Association's (ANA) president and executive director, she made a substantial contribution to the professionalisation of nursing (Butts & Rich, 2011). The significance of the nurse-patient connection as a therapeutic interpersonal process was highlighted in Peplau's groundbreaking work, Interpersonal Relations in Nursing (1952). She distinguished between four psychobiological experiences – needs, frustrations, conflicts, and anxieties – that elicit either positive or negative reactions in patients (Alligood, 2014a, 2018). The nurse-patient interaction may be divided into four phases, according to Peplau: orientation, identification, exploitation, and resolution. The stranger resource person, teacher, leader, surrogate, and counsellor are the six nursing roles that she suggested (Sills, 1998; Alligood, 2014a, 2018). The psychoanalytical model and the ideas of interpersonal relationships by Freud, Maslow, and Sullivan had an impact on her work. With recent publications focusing on staff-student relationships (Aghamohammadi-Kalkhoran et al., 2011; Alligood, 2014a, 2014b, 2018), psychiatric workforce development (Hanrahan et al., 2012; Alligood, 2014a, 2014b, 2018), attention-deficit/hyperactivity disorder care (Keoghan, 2011; Alligood, 2014a, 2014b, 2018), subject recruitment (Penckofer et al., 2011; Alligood, 2014a, 2014b, 2018), retention, and participation in research, and therapeutic relationships between women with anorexia and healthcare professionals (Wright & Hacking, 2012;

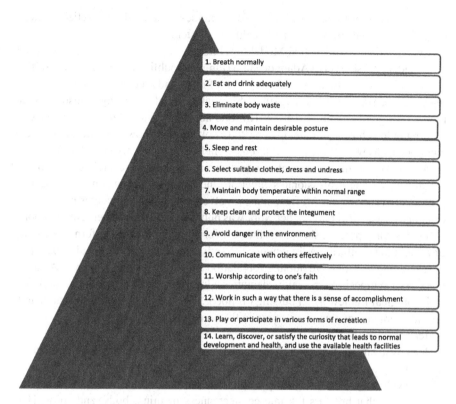

FIGURE 1.2   Henderson's basic needs (Henderson, 1991).

Alligood, 2014a, 2014b, 2018), her work on nurse-patient relationships continues to influence nursing practice and research.

Virginia Henderson (b.1897, d.1996):

Virginia Henderson, known as the "First Lady of Nursing", developed one of the most influential nursing theories (Henderson, 1955, 1960, 1966; Alligood, 2018), known as the "Henderson's Principles of Nursing" (see Figure 1.2) (Henderson, 1964, 1966; Alligood, 2018). Published in 1966, Henderson's theory emphasised the nurse's role in assisting individuals to achieve independence in meeting their basic needs (Henderson, 1966; Alligood, 2018).

Her definition of nursing as "assisting individuals to gain independence in activities of daily living" continues to guide nursing practice and education worldwide (Henderson, 1966, 1991; Alligood, 2018).

Paul Snelling (b.1925, d.2007):

Paul Snelling, a British nurse theorist, made significant contributions to nursing theory development in the latter half of the 20th century. His "Principles of Nursing Practice" framework emphasised the importance of individualised care, therapeutic communication, and evidence-based practice. Snelling's work highlighted the dynamic nature of nursing and the need for nurses to adapt their practice to meet the changing needs of patients and healthcare systems.

Evelyn Adam – Conceptual Model for Nursing

Canadian nurse Evelyn Adam began writing and publishing in the middle of the 1970s. Her research focuses on the creation of ideas and models related to the nursing concept (Adam, 1983, 1987, 1999). She makes use of a Dorothy Johnson-taught model (Alligood, 2014a, 2014b, 2018). She adapts Virginia Henderson's concept of nursing to Johnson's model in her 1980 book *To Be a Nurse*, identifying the key components as well as the presumptions, beliefs, and values (Adam, 1980).

Adam covers the purpose of the profession, the person receiving the professional service, the professional's function, the cause of the person receiving the professional service, the professional's involvement, and the outcomes in the latter category. A second version of her work was published in 1991. In her seminal book, "Modèles conceptuels", she makes the case for their significance in forming a style of thinking and offering a framework for activity (Adam, 1999). A solid example of leveraging a distinctive nursing foundation for future growth is seen in Adam's work. At a symposium on health telematics education, Adam presented his case for an ideological framework in nursing (Tallberg, 1997). She used prior research and provided concise explanations to aid in the construction of theories.

Jean Watson (b. 1940):

Jean Watson, an American nurse theorist, is renowned for her development of the "Theory of Human Caring". Grounded in existential philosophy and transpersonal psychology, Watson's theory emphasises the importance of holistic, compassionate care that honours the interconnectedness of mind, body, and spirit. Her framework has been widely adopted in nursing education and practice, promoting a culture of caring and healing in healthcare settings.

The development of nursing theory has been a dynamic and iterative process, driven by the visionary insights of nurse theorists throughout history. From Florence Nightingale's pioneering work in establishing nursing as a respected profession to modern theorists like Virginia Henderson, Paul Snelling, and Jean Watson, each has contributed to the rich tapestry of nursing knowledge and practice. Their theories continue to inform and inspire nurses worldwide, guiding the delivery of patient-centred, evidence-based care in an ever-changing healthcare landscape. These influential nurses have left an indelible mark on the nursing profession, inspiring generations of nurses to advocate for excellence in patient care, social justice, and public health. Their contributions continue to shape the future of nursing and advance the profession's commitment to promoting health and healing in diverse communities worldwide.

International perspectives

In recent years, the intersection of 'digital nursing' and nursing theory has gained prominence on a global scale, with organisations such as the World Health

Organization (WHO) and the International Council of Nurses (ICN) playing key roles in shaping policy, practice, and education. This following section explores international perspectives on digital nursing, focusing on the WHO Global Strategy, the ICN's position statement, and considerations for nursing scope of practice.

The World Health Organization (WHO) recognises the transformative potential of digital health technologies in improving access to quality healthcare and achieving universal health coverage. In 2021, the WHO released its Global Strategy on Digital Health, outlining a roadmap for harnessing the power of digital technologies to advance health outcomes worldwide. The strategy emphasises the importance of interoperable, scalable, and sustainable digital solutions that prioritise equity, inclusivity, and ethical considerations. Within the context of nursing, the WHO Global Strategy (2021) underscores the critical role of nurses in leveraging digital technologies to enhance patient care, promote health equity, and strengthen health systems. By embracing digital nursing competencies, nurses may contribute to the achievement of global health goals, including the Sustainable Development Goals (SDGs), through innovative approaches to service delivery, education, and research.

The International Council of Nurses (ICN), as the global voice of nursing, advocates for the advancement of nursing practice, education, and policy on the international stage. In its position statement on nursing and digital health, the International Council of Nurses (ICN) (2023) emphasises the importance of integrating digital technologies into nursing practice while upholding ethical standards, privacy rights, and patient confidentiality. The ICN (2023) recognises the potential of digital nursing to enhance patient safety, improve health outcomes, and facilitate interdisciplinary collaboration. However, it also acknowledges the need for ongoing education and training to ensure that nurses possess the necessary competencies to effectively utilise digital tools in their practice. Additionally, the ICN (2023) calls for policies that support nurses' engagement in the design, implementation, and evaluation of digital health solutions to ensure that they align with the needs and preferences of patients and communities.

As digital technologies continue to evolve, nurses must navigate new complex legal, ethical, and regulatory issues related to their scope of practice. The integration of digital nursing interventions, such as telehealth consultations, remote monitoring, and electronic documentation, requires careful consideration of jurisdictional regulations, professional standards, and liability concerns in addition to challenges to professional identity. Notably in a recent study by Wong et al. (2023), it was discovered that Australian nursing students may (unsurprisingly) have preconceptions about what nursing is when they enter the field, and these may not be compatible with digitally driven care processes. While some students were at ease with technology and could see how it will improve healthcare systems, many will be scared, nervous, and ill-prepared to utilise digital health technology. To create frameworks that allow students to use technology in conjunction with caregiving (Ali et al., 2022), simulation scenarios have the potential to improve students' ability to make decisions (O'Connor & LaRue, 2021) by stimulating novel perspectives on how workload, collaboration, and professional identity are portrayed in a digital health technology setting (Wong et al., 2023).

Ultimately, Wong et al. (2023) justify that a new understanding of what it means to be a nurse in the digital age has to be developed. This new understanding should preserve the special responsibilities of nurses while fostering DHT innovation to improve our ability to offer higher-quality, safer patient care. Nursing organisations and regulatory bodies play a crucial role in establishing guidelines and standards of practice for digital nursing within their respective jurisdictions. By clarifying nurses' roles, responsibilities, and competencies in the digital realm, these entities can promote safe, ethical, and effective use of technology in nursing care delivery.

In summary, international perspectives on digital nursing underscore the transformative potential of digital health technologies in advancing nursing practice, education, and policy on a global scale. Through collaboration, advocacy, and innovation, nurses can harness the power of digital technologies to improve health outcomes, promote health equity, and address the evolving needs of patients and communities worldwide.

Theories of nursing and digital technology

The significance of new technology and digital technology, in particular, is increasingly recognised as an issue which nurses must incorporate into their practice philosophies and professional identity. Evidence of this can be observed in recent calls for 'technology' itself to be considered a metaparadigm concept in nursing (Bayuo et al., 2023; Johnson & Carrington, 2023). Bayuo et al. (2023) proposed that technology be considered alongside the traditional metaparadigm domains of person, health, environment, and nursing. Utilising Fawcett's criteria for metaparadigm concepts, they consider the pervasive role of technology in nursing – spanning clinical practice, education, administration, and research – and argue that technology not only intersects with existing nursing domains but also adds a distinct, invaluable dimension to the discipline. The authors contend that technology, through its broad application and impact, satisfies the requirements of distinctiveness, encompassing phenomena of interest, perspective-neutrality, and international scope. This argument was further developed by Johnson and Carrington (2023) who consider the reality of modern humans, inseparable from technology, be this in the form of smartphones, wearable monitors, or implanted devices. This concept is consistent with the growing cultural acceptance of humans as 'cyborg' or the ongoing discourse around transhumanism. It is argued that nurses must incorporate these new concepts within the metaparadigm of the profession to stay relevant in the digital era and ensure that nursing's core human-focused goals remain achievable.

Contemporary nurse theorists have sought to explore key concepts in nursing including 'care', 'nursing presence', and relations between humans and robot technologies. Key examples of these contemporary theories can be seen in Table 1.2.

TABLE 1.2 Summary of theories relating to digital technology and nursing

Reference Country of Origin	Theory	Focus of Theory	Key Features/Premises
Abiko (1999) Japan	The nursing model of technology	The role of technology in society and nursing and how technology should be developed to support nursing	The theory posits that technology's role in the nursing context should facilitate managing the patient environment to promote health and assist patients in adapting to their surroundings. It advocates for a dynamic of 'intelligent obedience' between nurses (as technologists) and patients (as consumers), with a strong emphasis on placing patients at the forefront and ensuring informed consent in technology-related interactions.
Ji-Young et al. (2007) USA	The Information Communication Technology Acceptance Model (ICTAM)	Health consumers use of nursing informatics	The model introduces the Information and Communication Technology Acceptance Model (ICTAM), an evolution of the Technology Acceptance Model (TAM), to better reflect the specific ways health consumers utilise online resources to gather health information.
Locsin and Purnell (2015) USA	Technological competency as caring in nursing theory	The use of technology to support both caring and the preservation of humanness. This requires technological expertise	This perspective views individuals as part of a broader technological realm, suggesting that through technological proficiency, nurses can deliver care effectively.
Shankel and Wofford (2016) USA	Symptom Management Theory as a Clinical Practice Model for Symptom Telemonitoring in Chronic Disease	The use of telemedicine to manage patient symptoms remotely	Describes how patients' symptom experiences progress through various phases leading to 'symptom status outcomes', which can affect their quality of life, morbidity, or management of future symptoms. The application of telemonitoring can alter these phases, improving the likelihood of favourable symptom outcomes.

(Continued)

TABLE 1.2 (Continued)

Reference Country of Origin	Theory	Focus of Theory	Key Features/Premises
Barrett (2017) England	A grounded theory of nurses and teleconsultation	The use of teleconsultation technology by nurses	The theory outlines the crucial roles of nurses in telemedicine by emphasising 'being there' for patients through four types of presence: operational, clinical, social, and therapeutic.
Nagel et al. (2016) Canada	Getting a Picture: Nurses knowing the person in a virtual environment	How nurses come to 'know' patients when using remote patient monitoring	This approach suggests nurses construct a comprehensive understanding of their patients by integrating diverse data sources, necessitating advanced skills beyond traditional nursing education and the seamless integration of technology.
Tanioka (2017) Tanioka et al. (2019) Japan	The transactive relationship theory of nursing (TRETON): A nursing engagement model for persons and humanoid nursing robots	The relationship between human persons and humanoid nursing robots	Views nursing as an interplay between humans and intelligent machines, where nurses utilise technology in care practices, and some intelligent machines with artificial intelligence (AI) can simulate human interactions, highlighting the reliance on and ethical considerations of technology in nursing.
Bahari et al. (2021) Indonesia	Technological creativity as caring in nursing theory	The creation of nursing technologies as caring	The theory encourages active participation in the design of nursing technologies through collaboration with nurse-innovators, enhancing care delivery and refining the nursing process.

Source: Adapted from Wynn et al. (2023).

A synthesis of these theories was undertaken by Wynn et al. (2023) to identify key concepts consistent across these theories related to technology in nursing. This synthesis resulted in the Lens for Digital Nursing (LDN) which includes three broad concepts from which further theorising and research around digital technology in nursing might be undertaken. The key concepts include:

1 *Knowing the person* – the main function of the use of technologies by nurses to develop an understanding of aspects of an individual which guides clinical decision-making. This can be considered broadly to be what nurses use technology for.
2 *Technological competence* – the competence of nurses to operate, create, and appreciate both the limitations and ethical implications of technology in clinical contexts. This includes the person-centred use of technology to support nursing care. This can be considered broadly how nurses achieve knowing of the patient.
3 *Technology as an agent within the care environment* – the recognition by nurses that the presence or absence of technology can influence clinical outcomes due to its design or functionality. This can be considered broadly to be the reason nurses must interact with technologies. It also highlights the role of technology in augmenting the reach of nursing care in the absence of human nurses, for example, via the use of AI-driven robots, the user interfaces of digital platforms or highly integrated digital record systems.

It is proposed that these concepts are interconnected and can be used to explore nursing practices at both a macro patient-nurse level in addition to exploring nursing from a community or population perspective. Hence the 'Lens' can be zoomed in and out (Wynn et al., 2023). An example of this lens being used to explore potential new nursing practices in the context of communicable disease control can be seen in Chapter 6.

The rise of the digital patient

The phenomena of digital patients only exist within the reality of a digital society, and although this may seem obvious, it is important to explore notions of how digital interfaces are represented within populations. There are significant digital events that affect digital progression and proliferation, these include but are not limited to; the advent of the personal computer in the home, home-internet services, Wi-Fi, the launch of mobile devices and associated apps, the viral growth of social media, and more recently, wearable devices. According to Barnatt (2001), the digital revolution of the 1990s focused upon the transformation of media, products, and services into binary formats, with what he termed 'The Second Digital Revolution' theorised as mobile in nature with the potential for online methods of engagement. It is important to note that at the time of writing, Barnatt (2001) was years away from an iPhone or Facebook account.

The Second Digital Revolution is considered differently by Rindfleisch (2020) who has the benefit of hindsight in exploring the digital timeline; here, the first digital revolution is represented by the digitisation of goods via personal computers and the second focusing upon the opportunity to create goods at home with 3D printing. While this is a valid position, it does not acknowledge the significant impact of social media, especially the way that physical entities became not only visible in the digital world but also enabled interaction and trade.

These differences in the nuances of definitions and timelines for digital development and proliferation are an example of the nebulous nature of digital assimilation into everyday workplaces, homes, and recreational activities. Globally, these differences are amplified by digital accessibility to fundamental hardware: Traxler and Leach (2006) highlighted the physical constraints with infrastructure in Africa. It is useful to consider and recognise that the digital revolution encompassed a range of hardware and software developmental tipping points, assimilated rapidly and for the most part, driven by a consumerist agenda. Fundamentally, it is difficult to find an area of society that has not been touched by different digital technologies, however, there is an idea that some within the populations have surpassed purely digital approaches and are considered *postdigital*. In practice, such a position rarely reflects a definitive digital status and is instead represented by the ease of transition between digital and physical activities, such as reading, banking, or socialising with friends. Such activities are benign compared to ideas explored by Jandrić and Hayes (2023): their exploration of post-digitalism is based on futurology and a 'social science fiction'.

In this fiction, the biotech industry provides a foundation for technological innovations that seem as incredible as they are implausible, that is until the comparison is made with a company based in the US that has developed a brain-computer interface and is running clinical trials.

Defining the digital patient

The impact of digital proliferation is difficult to measure or fully understand, nevertheless, there are indications of influence within business, politics, and healthcare.

Malone et al. (2005) offered an early idea of what a digital patient could be, reflective of the technologies of the time and challenging the traditional notion of the patient-doctor relationship. Their research found a distinct typology, separate from traditional approaches to seeking health information; such patients were entitled 'information hungry'/ 'online' health seekers. This phenomenon is important when exploring ideas of the digital patient and marks a shift in not only the relationship between patient and doctor but also sets in motion a position of individual responsibility and the possibility of using digital approaches to research, measure, and share personal health data.

Since that time, all patients or service users will have had a level of digital presence, regardless of their own views on the matter; digitised medical and nursing notes, including medical images are the norm in many developed healthcare economies. Many will have had their symptoms entered into an algorithm when calling for telephone advice and it is likely that for some, Artificial Intelligence has either helped with their diagnosis or been involved in the planning of their care. In this instance, the term *passive digital patient* could be used to describe those who, for the most part, are not digitally engaged themselves, but through their interactions, have their personal health data translated into digital entities.

The juxtaposition of the passive are those who are *active digital patients*; they also reflect the experience of *passive digital patients,* where the enrolment into digital systems is the foundation and entry point to many worldwide healthcare economies. However, *active digital patients* go further and invest in hardware, software or embrace digital communities that impact upon health choices, and they may do so embracing and advocating the technology, or instead, with a *postdigital bent,* without mention or even the perception that their actions are based in a metaphysical digital domain.

The way technology is embraced and used for active digital patients is as diverse as the technology they use; variations include the measurement of some vital signs, tracking steps or cadence, logging daily calorific or nutrient intake, blood glucose monitoring, menstruation tracking, sleep quality, vaccine records, and medical notes. One commonality that most active digital patients share is that most of the daily management of technology occurs through the auspices of 'apps' on a mobile device, often, a mobile or smartphone. Such devices, connected to wearables or appliances within the home, workplace, or leisure environments help to manage and present the mass amounts of data collected, building a complex picture of the individual behaviours impacting upon health.

On a spectrum (see Figure 1.3) of digital use, passive and active patients manifest within a field of common attributes, there exist bipolar extremes of digital atavism

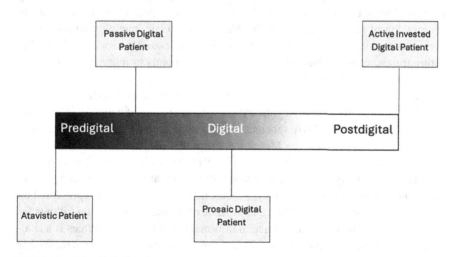

FIGURE 1.3   The digital patient spectrum.

and digitally invested patients, aligning to ideas of pre-digital and postdigital existence. The middle ground can be considered to be a place of everyday practice, where people neither protest nor promote a digital position.

Patient education and digital health literacy

In a digital or postdigital world, where information and access to personal data relating to health has been at least partially democratised, there is an opportunity to consider this position against health outcomes. There is global consensus that reaching a step count of 10,000 steps per day helps to attain a level of health benefit for both physical and mental health. The measurement of step-counts is not a new phenomenon, and commercial, inexpensive pedometers have long been available. This poses the question of why specific wearables and their associated apps are chosen over the original pedometers. It can be postulated that those invested within digital health solutions see some extra benefit in the presentation and storage of data and the further range of metrics collected. The addition of competitive tournaments might also be an incentive for some, such as micro-credential 'digital badges'.

There is likely a discourse of credibility associated with certain digital health tools that are not found in similar products in the physical world. For years, and for a fee, community-based weight loss *clubs* have offered dietary advice, often based upon calorific reduction and group support, however, these may not be comfortable experiences for all. The digital representation of this is free, enables easy tracking of caloric intake and links to other fitness apps; the process is individualised, even setting personal goals for nutrient intakes. Maybe, going digital in this area is seen as more credible and dare it be said, 'of the moment'. While perceptions of *coolness* or trend may seem kitsch to some, it is significant to note that in the postdigital world, both digital and physical representation are equally important and engaging in technologies of the moment can form part of this representation. The ultimate progression of personalised digital health is likely to continue with consumer-led service expansion and proliferation and while it is impossible to accurately predict future trends, consideration of past developments points to more personal health data being accessible to digital patients.

The advent of the SARS-COV-2 virus and the subsequent COVID-19 pandemic amplified and fuelled conspiracy theories around the nature of zoonotic viruses and their treatments with mRNA vaccines. Such a conspiracy in the UK appeared in the *Lancet* in 1998, where the Measles, Mumps, and Rubella vaccine was linked to autism and bowel disease (Godlee et al., 2011) by Andrew Wakefield et al. The research was quickly discredited; however, the ramification of this research likely underpins current vaccine hesitancy, a factor that was significantly represented on many online social media platforms at the time of the mass vaccination rollouts for SARS-COV-2. The validation of health information from digital sources is a challenge for both patients and nurses alike and there is likely a requirement for further consideration at the policy level. Understanding why people believe and accept conspiracy while rejecting peer-reviewed research-based health information, and the influence that some digital entities hold over others when making health decisions is a serious risk to overall population health. Advances in vaccine technology mean that the world is facing a new future where the prevalence of some diseases is forever changed; like Smallpox, Polio could be wiped from modern memory worldwide (Bhaumik, 2012). Likewise, the HPV vaccine reduces cervical cancer incidence by up to 87% (Falcaro et al., 2021). Such miraculous biotechnology advances are testament to the human spirit of endeavour; however, such innovation will serve to be a lesson in futility only, unless digital patients develop ideas of verisimilitude. Crucially, whether passive or active, modern nurses must recognise the inherent 'digital-ness' of their patients; a concept emphasised by contemporary scholarship calling for technology itself to be recognised as a nursing metaparadigm concept. To understand our patients' personhood, health, and environment, nursing practices must adapt to account for the digitalisation of life more broadly.

Chapter summary

This chapter has explored the multifaceted nature of the nursing profession, tracing its historical origins, evolution, and the significant impact of technological advancements on nursing practices and education. It began by delineating nursing's roots, highlighting its essential role in human societies and the transition from informal caregiving roles, largely undertaken by women, to a more structured and formalised profession through the pioneering efforts of Florence Nightingale among others. The establishment of the first official school of nursing marked a crucial step in professionalising nursing, emphasising both theoretical education and practical experience.

The chapter further examined the challenges of defining the nursing profession, noting the lack of a precise definition even as nursing education and registration became formalised. This ambiguity has led to debates around the professional identity of nurses and the role of ritualistic practices in nursing care. The advent of digital technologies was identified as a double-edged sword, offering opportunities to enhance patient care while also threatening to depersonalise care through the digitisation of traditional nursing practices. A critical discussion on nursing as a socio-political assemblage underscored the influence of socio-political factors on nursing practices and the profession's struggle to maintain its distinctiveness amid shifting healthcare roles. The chapter argued for a critical re-evaluation of nursing education and practice, advocating for a pedagogical shift towards empowering nurses to make unique contributions to healthcare.

Theoretical developments in nursing were explored, from the foundational contributions of Nightingale to contemporary theorists who have sought to integrate digital technology into nursing paradigms. These developments reflect nursing's ongoing effort to articulate its scope, ethical foundations, and practice standards in response to societal and technological changes.

Finally, the chapter addressed the emergence of the "digital patient" and the implications for nursing practice and patient care in the digital age. It highlighted the need for nurses to develop digital competencies and engage critically with digital technologies to enhance care delivery while preserving the profession's core values of patient-centred care.

References

Abiko, S. (1999). Lessons from nursing theories: Toward the humanisation of technology. *AI and Society, 13*(1–2), 164–175. doi:10.1007/BF01205265

Adam, E. (1980). *To be a nurse*. Philadelphia: Saunders.

Adam, E. (1983). Frontiers of nursing in the 21st century: Development of models and theories on the concept of nursing. *Journal of Advanced Nursing, 8*, 41–45.

Adam, E. (1987). Nursing theory: What it is and what it is not. *Nursing Papers. Perspectives in Nursing, 19*, 5–14.

Adam, E. (1999). Conceptual models. *Canadian Journal of Nursing Research, 30*, 103–114.

Aghamohammadi-Kalkhoran, M., Karimollahi, M., & Abdi, R. (2011). Iranian staff nurses' attitudes toward nursing students. *Nurse Education Today, 31*, 477–481.

Ali, S., Kleib, M., Paul, P., Petrovskaya, O., & Kennedy, M. (2022). Compassionate nursing care and the use of digital health technologies: A scoping review. *International Journal of Nursing Studies, 127*, 104161. doi:10.1016/j.ijnurstu.2021.104161

Alligood, M. R. (2004). Nursing theory: The basis for professional nursing practice. In K. K. Chitty (Ed.), *Professional nursing: Concepts and challenges* (4th ed., pp. 271–298). Philadelphia: Saunders.

Alligood, M. R. (2010a). The nature of knowledge needed for nursing practice. In M. R. Alligood (Ed.), *Nursing theory: Utilization & application* (4th ed., pp. 3–15). St. Louis: Mosby.

Alligood, M. R. (2010b). Models and theories: Critical thinking structures. In M. R. Alligood (Ed.), *Nursing theory: Utilization & application* (4th ed., pp. 43–65). St. Louis: Mosby.

Alligood, M. R. (2014a). *Nursing theorists and their work*. Elsevier.

Alligood, M. R. (2014b). *Nursing theory: Utilization & application* (5th ed.). Maryland Heights: Mosby-Elsevier.

Alligood, M. R. (2018). *Nursing theorists and their work*. Elsevier.

Alligood, M. R., & Tomey, A. M. (Eds.). (1997). *Nursing theory: Utilization & application*. St. Louis: Mosby.

Alligood, M. R., & Tomey, A. M. (Eds.). (2010). *Nursing theorists and their work* (7th ed.). Maryland Heights: Mosby-Elsevier.

Bahari, K., Talosig, A. T., & Pizarro, J. B. (2021). Nursing technologies creativity as an expression of caring: A grounded theory study. *Global Qualitative Nursing Research, 8*, 2333393621997397. doi:10.1177/2333393621997397

Barnatt, C. (2001). The second digital revolution. *Journal of General Management, 27*(2), 1–16.

Barrett, D. (2017). Rethinking presence: A grounded theory of nurses and teleconsultation. *Journal of Clinical Nursing, 26*(19–20), 3088–3098. doi:10.1111/jocn.13656

Batey, M. V. (1977). Conceptualization: Knowledge and logic guiding empirical research. *Nursing Research, 26*(5), 324–329.

Bauman, Z. (1991). The social manipulation of morality: Moralizing actors, adiaphorizing action. *Theory, Culture & Society, 8*(1), 137–151. doi:10.1177/026327691008001007

Bayuo, J., Abu-Odah, H., Su, J. J., & Aziato, L. (2023). Technology: A metaparadigm concept of nursing. *Nursing Inquiry, 30*(4), e12592. doi:10.1111/nin.12592

Bender, M. (2018). Re-conceptualizing the nursing metaparadigm: Articulating the philosophical ontology of the nursing discipline that orients inquiry and practice. *Nursing Inquiry, 25*(3), e12243. doi:10.1111/nin.12243

Bhaumik, S. (2012). Polio eradication: Current status and challenges. *Journal of Family Medicine and Primary Care, 1*(2), 84–85. doi:10.4103/2249-4863.104936. PMID: 24479012; PMCID: PMC3893965.

Bixler, G. K., & Bixler, R. W. (1959). The professional status of nursing. *American Journal of Nursing, 59*(8), 1142–1146.

Blackburn, J., Ousey, K., & Stephenson, J. (2019). Nurses' education, confidence, and competence in appropriate dressing choice. *Advances in Skin & Wound Care, 32*(10), 470–476. doi:10.1097/01.ASW.0000577132.81124.88

Butts, J. B., & Rich, K. L. (2011). *Philosophies and theories for advanced nursing practice.* Sudbury: Jones & Bartlett.

Chinn, P. L., & Kramer, M. K. (2011). *Integrated knowledge development in nursing* (8th ed.). St. Louis: Elsevier Mosby.

Collier-Sewell, F., Atherton, I., Mahoney, C., Kyle, R. G., Hughes, E., & Lasater, K. (2023). Competencies and standards in nurse education: The irresolvable tensions. *Nurse Education Today, 125*, 105782. doi:10.1016/j.nedt.2023.105782

Davies, C. (1995). *Gender and the professional predicament in nursing.* Great Britain: Open University Press.

Draper, J. (1985). Make the dressing fit the wound. *Nursing Times, 81*(41), 32–34.

Egenes, K. (2017). *History of nursing in issues and trends in nursing, practice, policy and leadership.* Jones & Bartlett Learning.

Falcaro, M., Castañon, A., Ndlela, B., Checchi, M., Soldan, K., & Lopez-Bernal, J. (2021). The effects of the national HPV vaccination programme in England, UK, on cervical cancer and grade 3 cervical intraepithelial neoplasia incidence: A register-based observational study. *The Lancet, 398*(10316), 2084–2092.

Fawcett, J. (1978). The relationship between theory and research: A double helix. *Advances in Nursing Science, 1*(1), 49–62.

Fawcett, J. (1984). The metaparadigm of nursing: Present status and future refinements. *Image: The Journal of Nursing Scholarship, 16*(3), 84–87. doi:10.1111/j.1547-5069.1984.tb01393.x

Fawcett, J. (1993). *Analysis and evaluation of nursing theories.* Philadelphia: F. A. Davis.

Fawcett, J. (2005). *Contemporary nursing knowledge: Conceptual models of nursing and nursing theories* (2nd ed.). Philadelphia: F. A. Davis.

Fawcett, J., & Garity, J. (2009). *Evaluating research for evidence-based nursing practice.* Philadelphia: F.A.Davis.

Fitzpatrick, J., & Whall, A. (1983). *Conceptual models of nursing.* Bowie: Robert J. Brady.

Freire, P., & Ramos, M. B. (1996). *Pedagogy of the oppressed* (Rev. ed.). Penguin.

Gauci, P., Luck, L., O'Reilly, K., & Peters, K. (2023). Workplace gender discrimination in the nursing workforce—An integrative review. *Journal of Clinical Nursing, 32*, 5693–5711. doi:10.1111/jocn.16684

Godlee, F., Smith, J., & Marcovitch, H. (2011). Wakefield's article linking MMR vaccine and autism was fraudulent. *BMJ, 2011*, 342, c7452 doi:10.1136/bmj.c7452

Guest, J. F., Fuller, G. W., & Vowden, P. (2020). Cohort study evaluating the burden of wounds to the UK's National Health Service in 2017/2018: Update from 2012/2013. *BMJ Open, 10*, e045253. doi:10.1136/bmjopen-2020-045253

Hanrahan, N. P., Delaney, D., & Stuart, G. W. (2012). Blueprint for development of the advanced practice psychiatric nurse workforce. *Nursing Outlook, 60*, 91–106.

Hardy, M. E. (1974). Theories: Components, development, evaluation. *Nursing Research, 23*(2), 100–107.

Henderson, V. (1955). *Textbook of the principles and practice of nursing* (5th ed.). New York: Macmillan (Note: earlier editions were Harmer & Henderson).

Henderson, V. (1960). *Basic principles of nursing care*. London: International Council of Nurses.

Henderson, V. (1964). The nature of nursing. *American Journal of Nursing, 64*, 62–68.

Henderson, V. (1966). *The nature of nursing: A definition and its implications for practice, research, and education*. New York: Macmillan.

Henderson, V. (1980). Preserving the essence of nursing in a technological age. *Journal of Advanced Nursing, 5*, 245–260.

Henderson, V. A. (1991). *The nature of nursing: Reflections after 25 years*. New York: National League for Nursing Press.

Holliday, M. E., & Parker, D. L. (1997). Florence Nightingale, feminism and nursing. *Journal of Advanced Nursing, 26*, 483–488. doi:10.1046/j.1365-2648.1997.t01-6-00999.x

Im, E. O., & Chang, S. J. (2012). Current trends in nursing theories. *Journal of Nursing Scholarship, 44*(2), 156–164.

International Council of Nurses (ICN) (2023). The future of nursing and digital health: New ICN position statement highlights opportunities and risks. Retrieved from https://www.icn.ch/news/future-nursing-and-digital-health-new-icn-position-statement-highlights-opportunities-and-risks [Accessed 25.2.24].

Jandrić, P., & Hayes, S. (2023). Postdigital education in a biotech future. *Policy Futures in Education, 21*(5), 503–513. doi:10.1177/14782103211049915

Ji-Young, A., Hayman, L. L., Panniers, T., Carty, B., & An, J.-Y. (2007). Theory development in nursing and healthcare informatics: A model explaining and predicting information and communication technology acceptance by healthcare consumers. *ANS, 30*(3), E37–E49. doi:10.1097/01.ANS.0000286628.92386.40

Johnson, E., & Carrington, J. M. (2023). Revisiting the nursing metaparadigm: Acknowledging technology as foundational to progressing nursing knowledge. *Nursing Inquiry, 30*(1), e12502. doi:10.1111/nin.12502

Kalisch, P. A., & Kalisch, B. J. (2003). *American nursing: A history* (4th ed.). Philadelphia: Lippincott.

Keoghan, S. (2011). Attention deficit hyperactivity disorder: A model of nursing care. *Mental Health Practice, 215*, 20–22.

Kuhn, T. S. (1970). *The structure of scientific revolutions*. Chicago: University of Chicago Press.

Locsin, R. C., & Purnell, M. (2015). Advancing the theory of technological competency as caring in nursing: The universal technological domain. *International Journal for Human Caring, 19*(2), 50–54.

Malone, M., Mathes, L., Dooley, J., & While, A. E. (2005). Health information seeking and its effect on the doctor-patient digital divide. *Journal of Telemedicine and Telecare, 11*(1_suppl), 25–28. doi:10.1258/1357633054461831

McCarthy, M. P., & Jones, J. S. (2019). The medicalization of nursing: The loss of a discipline's unique identity. *International Journal for Human Caring, 23*(1). doi:10.20467/1091-5710.23.1.101

Meleis, A. (2007). *Theoretical nursing: Development and progress* (4th ed.). Philadelphia: Lippincott.

Nagel, D. A., Stacey, D., Momtahan, K., Gifford, W., Doucet, S., & Etowa, J. B. (2016). Getting a picture: A grounded theory of nurses knowing the person in a virtual environment. *Journal of Holistic Nursing, 35*(1), 67–85. doi:10.1177/0898010116645422

Nicoll, L. (1986). *Perspectives on nursing theory*. Boston: Little, Brown.

Nicoll, L. (1992). *Perspectives on nursing theory* (2nd ed.). Philadelphia: Lippincott, Williams & Wilkins.

Nicoll, L. (1997). *Perspectives on nursing theory* (3rd ed.). Philadelphia: Lippincott, Williams & Wilkins.

Nightingale, F. (1969). *Notes on nursing: What it is and what it is not*. New York: Dover (Originally published in 1859).

O'Connor, S., & LaRue, E. (2021). Integrating informatics into undergraduate nursing education: A case study using a spiral learning approach. *Nurse Education in Practice, 50,* 102934. doi:10.1016/j.nepr.2020.102934

Paley, J. (2002). Caring as a slave morality: Nietzschean themes in nursing ethics. *Journal of Advanced Nursing, 40*(1), 25–35. doi:10.1046/j.1365-2648.2002.02337.x

Parker, M. (2006). *Nursing theory and nursing practice* (2nd ed.). Philadelphia: F. A. Davis.

Penckofer, S., Byrn, M., Mumby, P., & Ferrans, C. E. (2011). Improving subject recruitment, retention, and participation in research through Peplau's theory of interpersonal relations. *Nursing Science Quarterly, 24,* 146–151.

Peplau, H. E. (1952). *Interpersonal relations in nursing*. New York: Putnam.

Peterson, S. (2008). *Middle-range theories: Applications to nursing research* (2nd ed.). Philadelphia: Lippincott, Williams & Wilkins.Reed, P., & Shearer, N. (2009). *Perspectives on nursing theory* (5th ed.). New York: Lippincott Williams & Wilkins.

Reed, P., & Shearer, N. (2012). *Perspectives on nursing theory* (6th ed.). New York: Lippincott Williams & Wilkins.

Reed, P., Shearer, N., & Nicoll, L. (2003). *Perspectives on nursing theory* (4th ed.). Philadelphia: Lippincott, Williams & Wilkins.

Rindfleisch, A. (2020). The second digital revolution. *Marketing Letters, 2020*(31), 13–17.

Rubeis, G. (2023). Adiaphorisation and the digital nursing gaze: Liquid surveillance in long-term care. *Nursing Philosophy, 24,* e12388. doi:10.1111/nup.12388

Shankel, E. C., & Wofford, L. G. (2016). Symptom management theory as a clinical practice model for symptom telemonitoring in chronic disease. *Journal of Theory Construction & Testing, 10*(1), 31–38.

Sills, G. M. (1998). Peplau and professionalism: The emergence of the paradigm of professionalization. *Journal of Psychiatric and Mental Health Nursing, 5,* 167–171.

Specht, J. P., Bergquist, S., & Franz, R. A. (1995) Adoption of a research-based practice for treatment of pressure ulcers. *Nurse Clinics of North America, 30*(3), 553–563.

Smith, G., Greenwood, M., & Searle, R. (2010). Ward nurses' use of wound dressings before and after a bespoke education programme. *Journal of Wound Care, 19*(9), 396–402.

Smith, M., & Leihr, P. (2008). *Middle range theory for nursing* (2nd ed.). New York: Springer.

Tallberg, M. (1997). Supporting the nursing process—An aim for education in nursing informatics. In J. Mantas (Ed.), *Health telematics education: Studies in health technology and informatics* (vol 41, pp. 291–296). Amsterdam: IOS Press.

Tanioka, T. (2017). The development of the Transactive Relationship Theory of Nursing (TRETON): A nursing engagement model for persons and humanoid nursing robots. *International Journal of Nursing & Clinical Practices, 2017,* 1–8.

Tanioka, T., Yasuhara, Y., Dino, M. J. S., Kai, Y., Locsin, R. C., & Schoenhofer, S. O. (2019). Disruptive engagements with technologies, robotics, and caring: Advancing the Transactive Relationship Theory of Nursing. *Nursing Administration Quarterly, 43*(4), 313–321.

Thorne, S. (2023). On the misguided search for a definition of nursing. In *Nursing inquiry* (Vol. 30, Issue 4). Wiley. doi:10.1111/nin.12610

Traxler, J., & Leach, J. (2006). Innovative and sustainable mobile learning in Africa. In *2006 Fourth IEEE International Workshop on Wireless, Mobile and Ubiquitous Technology in Education (WMTE '06)*, Athens, Greece, pp. 98–102. doi:10.1109/WMTE.2006.261354

Walker, L. O., & Avant, K. C. (2011). *Strategies for theory construction in nursing* (5th ed.). Boston: Prentice Hall.

Wong, P., Brand, G., Dix, S., Choo, D., Foley, P., & Lokmic-Tomkins, Z. (2023). Pre-registration nursing students' perceptions of digital health technology on the future of nursing: A qualitative exploratory study. *Nurse Educator*, December 25, 2023. doi:10.1097/NNE.0000000000001591

Wood, A. F. (2010). Nursing models: Normal science for nursing practice. In M. R. Alligood (Ed.), *Nursing theory: Utilization & application* (4th ed., pp. 17–46). Maryland Heights: Mosby-Elsevier.

World Health Organization (WHO). (2021). Global strategy on digital health 2020–2025. Geneva: World Health Organization; 2021. Licence: CC BY-NC-SA 3.0 IGO. Retrieved from https://www.who.int/docs/default-source/documents/gs4dhdaa2a9f352b0445bafb c79ca799dce4d.pdf 25/02/2024

Wright, K. M., & Hacking, S. (2012). An angel on my shoulder: A study of relationships between women with anorexia and health care professionals. *Journal of Psychiatric and Mental Health Nursing, 19*, 107–112.

Wynn, M., Garwood-Cross, L., Vasilica, C., & Davis, D. (2023). Digital nursing practice theory: A scoping review and thematic analysis. *Journal of Advanced Nursing, 79*(11), 4137–4148. doi:10.1111/jan.15660

Ziebland, S., Hyde, E., & Powell, J. (2021). Power, paradox and pessimism: On the unintended consequences of digital health technologies in primary care. *Social Science & Medicine, 289*, 114419. doi:10.1016/j.socscimed.2021.114419

2

THE EVOLVING ROLE OF NURSES IN THE DIGITAL AGE

Cristina Vasilica, Neil Withnell and Joshi Prabhu Navis

Introduction

In today's rapidly advancing digital landscape, the role of nurses is undergoing a significant transformation. The integration of digital technologies into healthcare extends far beyond the mere adoption of new tools; it involves a profound reshaping of nursing care practices and processes. Traditionally seen as providers of direct patient care, nurses are now at the forefront of incorporating digital technologies into healthcare settings. From medical devices to electronic health records (EHRs), telehealth, and broader digital health platforms, these technologies are revolutionising how nurses deliver care, access evidence-based information, communicate with patients, and collaborate with other healthcare professionals.

Successful technology integration in nursing is not primarily reliant on the technology itself, but on the social context in which it is employed. For example, while the implementation of EHRs can streamline documentation and enhance patient outcomes, it also necessitates changes in workflow, training, and organisational culture. Nurses play a pivotal role in this process, as their feedback and interaction with new technologies are essential for ensuring both the effectiveness and acceptance of these tools. As the landscape of healthcare shifts, nurses are not merely passive recipients of these tools, but rather key agents in their implementation and optimisation. Their ability to adapt and influence workflows in response to new digital technologies sets the stage for a broader discussion of nursing informatics and the transformative potential it holds for patient care and professional practice.

The concept of digital technologies and society being co-constructed (Bijker et al., 2012) highlights how digital nursing transformation and social practices continually influence one another. This dynamic interplay is particularly evident in digital nursing, where the integration of technological tools not only transforms

DOI: 10.4324/9781032714547-2

nursing practices but also evolves in response to societal health needs, norms, and the rise of digital citizenship. In this context, researchers have called for a paradigm shift in both nursing science and practice (Pickler & Dorsey, 2021; Wong et al., 2023).

Over the past few decades, the field of informatics has driven a significant paradigm shift globally, advancing nursing roles that focus on managing data, information, and knowledge to support decision-making for patients, nurses, and other healthcare providers (Staggers, 2002). The rapid evolution of digital and social media has driven societal changes that significantly impact how individuals' access, interact with, and communicate health information. Social media platforms, smartphone applications, and health-tracking technology have disrupted traditional relationships between medical expert authority and lay health knowledge. Through social networks, patients now have access to vast health information and peer support, making them more informed and actively involved in their healthcare decisions (Vasilica, 2015; Vasilica & Ormandy, 2017; Vasilica et al., 2021). Consequently, patient expectations have become more informed and personalised, influencing healthcare systems to adopt innovative approaches to meet these evolving demands. This shift has led to a re-evaluation of the boundaries between non-specialist and specialist knowledge within healthcare and medical science (Hardey, 1999). This shift in patient knowledge and autonomy not only affects the patient-provider relationship but also requires nurses to adjust their roles within healthcare teams. The next section delves into the evolution of nursing informatics as a bridge between traditional nursing practice and the emerging demands of a more digitally engaged patient population

In this context, advancing digital nursing requires a paradigm shift in understanding nursing care in the digital age. This chapter explores the evolving role of nurses within this digital landscape, using the framework of Science and Technology Studies (STS). An STS approach allows the authors to examine the interplay between technological advancements and social practices, emphasising how nurses adapt to and influence these changes. By analysing the integration of digital tools such as EHRs, telemedicine, and health-tracking devices into nursing workflows, this chapter highlights how nurses' roles are being redefined. It also delves into the implications for patient care and professional development. Additionally, this discussion addresses the challenges and opportunities arising from this digital transformation, offering insights into how nurses can navigate and contribute to the evolving healthcare landscape.

Nursing informatics – a short history

The integration of technology in nursing has consistently evolved, marked by profound changes over the years. From measuring basic biometrics, like temperature, to more advanced therapeutic treatments, technology has played a pivotal role in shaping care. One simple example is the shift from mercury thermometers to digital thermometers, eliminating the risks posed by the neurotoxic effects of mercury and making temperature measurement more efficient. This shift, while seemingly straightforward, illustrates a fundamental transformation in how nurses collect, manage, and interpret data. Previously, nurses used mercury thermometers manually, which required time, skill, and careful attention to detail. Any delay or inaccuracy in recording temperatures could impact patient care. In contrast, digital thermometers allow for instant data collection and integration with electronic health systems (EHRs), improving speed and accuracy. The non-digital nature of mercury thermometers required nurses to record and track data manually, often leading to increased opportunities for human error. Now, the digitisation of these devices highlights the role of informatics in minimising such risks, making nursing practice more data-driven and efficient. Moreover, digital systems allow for longitudinal tracking of patient data, enabling nurses to identify trends and act more proactively in patient care. Similarly, manual mercury sphygmomanometers (used for measuring blood pressure) have been replaced by digital versions (Nimmagadda et al., 2018). Medical equipment has also advanced from early electronic devices to more sophisticated monitoring and imaging technologies, such as pacemakers, implantable devices, and minimally invasive surgical tools.

These technological advancements have expanded the scope of nursing practice, enabling nurses to collaborate more effectively with physicians in developing treatment plans and providing patients with more accurate information and support. Nurses have had to develop new expertise in managing patients with these technologies, educating them on faster recovery processes, and adapting to innovations that require ongoing professional development and specialised training. As information technology became integrated into various disciplines and social contexts, the term 'informatics' emerged to denote these intersections, leading to fields like medical informatics, health informatics, and business informatics. In 1980, Scholes and Barber introduced this concept to nursing, as 'nursing informatics' (Scholes & Barber, 1980). Over the years, this concept has continued to evolve as digital technologies became an integral part of nursing practice. The shift from, for example, mercury-based, analogue tools to digital instruments serves as a microcosm of the broader changes within nursing. It highlights the increasing reliance on real-time data, the reduction of manual processes, and the transformation of nursing from a hands-on, manually driven profession to one deeply intertwined with digital systems. These shifts are crucial for understanding how the role of nurses has expanded in scope, requiring not only bedside care but also a nuanced understanding of digital tools, data management, and the ability to engage in higher-level clinical decision-making processes.

The digital and technological dependence that has become integral to nursing care has transformed how nurses manage patient care and interact with other healthcare professionals. The integration of digital tools into nursing practice has been gradual but transformative. Alongside the broader digitisation of healthcare, nursing informatics began to evolve. A review of nursing informatics reveals three key themes for analysis: information technology–oriented, conceptually oriented, and role-oriented definitions (Staggers, 2002). The technology-centric view of nursing informatics emphasised the role of technology in collecting, storing, processing, and communicating data to support nursing functions across healthcare settings (Zielstorff et al., 1989; Hannah et al., 2006). However, this technology-centric approach faced criticism for overlooking essential non-digital informatics activities, such as the interplay between nurses, data, and care processes (Staggers, 2002). With these initial steps laying the foundation, the evolution of nursing informatics over the decades highlights a growing need for conceptual shifts. As we move from a purely technical understanding towards a more holistic, patient-centred approach, the boundaries of what it means to practice nursing are continuously being redefined

By the mid-1980s, nursing informatics began to shift from a technology-focused perspective to a more conceptually oriented one, although this change was not widely accepted until nearly 1990. The conceptually oriented approach expanded to include nursing-related information, goals, and the use of computers, all interconnected (Schwirian, 1989). This shift further defined nursing informatics as a combination of computer science, information science, and nursing science, aimed at managing nursing data, information, and knowledge (Graves & Corcoran-Perry, 1996). This new perspective downplayed the role of technology, aligning nursing informatics more closely with nursing practice and decision-making (Staggers, 2002).

In the late 1980s, particularly in the US, informatics nurse specialists became increasingly prevalent. These roles often required self-taught skills, focusing on integrating computer technology into healthcare settings. This led to a new definition of nurse informaticists by the American Nurses Association, which highlighted their role in managing data and information to support nursing functions and expand nursing knowledge. Despite this, the role-oriented approach did not gain widespread attention at the time (Staggers, 2002). The growing prevalence of these roles highlights a pivotal moment in nursing history, where nurses began to transition from being caregivers to becoming key players in the digitalisation of healthcare systems. However, this transformation was not without its challenges, as discussed in the emerging debates around technology-centred versus conceptually oriented definitions of nursing informatics.

As the field continued to develop, a greater focus on the patient began to emerge. Nursing informatics started to be recognised as a tool for decision-making by patients, nurses, and healthcare providers through information structures, processes, and technology, with the ultimate goal of improving health outcomes (Staggers, 2002). More recently, a narrative review identified over 14 definitions of nursing informatics, with Australia, the US, and Canada having the oldest documented definitions in the literature (Reid et al., 2021). The review emphasised the need for a global, unified stance on nursing informatics to provide nurses with a clearer understanding of the field. This would help create a consolidated body of knowledge, a defined educational mandate, and a digitally prepared workforce (Reid et al., 2021). Nurse informaticists play critical roles in improving workflow, facilitating communication between IT and nursing, and increasing the acceptance of clinical systems in healthcare (Sipes, 2019).

Despite the ambiguity surrounding the evolving role of nursing informatics in light of rapid technological advancements, existing concepts remain focused on data, information, and knowledge in nursing practice, all of which are supported by information structures, processes, and technology. In theory, nurse informaticists bridge the gap between clinical practice and information technology, ensuring that healthcare systems are designed and implemented to meet the needs of nurses and improve patient outcomes. They also play a vital role in educating and preparing the nursing workforce to effectively use technology in practice.

Technologies linked to health informatics encompass a wide range of tools and systems designed to manage, process, and analyse health-related data. These technologies are collectively referred to as Health Information Technologies (HITs) or technological components used for the storage, retrieval, analysis, and communication of health-related data (Neame et al., 2020). HITs play a crucial role in various healthcare processes, including managing patient records, scheduling essential interventions, communicating health information, and analysing data to support clinical decision-making (Neame et al., 2020). They include technologies such as electronic health records (EHRs), tools that enable remote healthcare services, and medical devices.

Clinical Decision Support Systems (CDSS) represent advanced health information technologies designed to assist clinicians in making informed decisions at the point of care. These systems provide clinicians, including nurses, with knowledge and patient-specific information to inform their practice. CDSS tools encompass computerised alerts and reminders, clinical guidelines, condition-specific order sets, patient data reports, documentation templates, diagnostic support, and contextually relevant reference materials. Knowledge-based systems use rules derived from clinical guidelines and existing evidence to make recommendations, while non-knowledge-based systems employ statistical analysis tools or machine learning algorithms to analyse large datasets, often gathered from EHRs, to generate insights (Dowding, 2024).

As these tools become more deeply embedded into clinical workflows, the role of nurses shifts from data entry and documentation towards more analytical and decision-support functions. This shift requires a re-evaluation of how we train nurses and what skills they need to navigate this new, data-driven healthcare environment.

Health information systems (HIS) are socio-technical subsystems within healthcare settings that encompass the entire data management ecosystem, including the policies, processes, and people involved (Winter et al., 2023). HIS functions range from EHRs to administrative registers, reminders, and illness management solutions across a variety of care settings, including academic medical centres, hospitals, clinics, general practices, laboratories, and patient homes (Lau et al., 2010). HIS acknowledges the mutual shaping of human and technical actors involved in these processes (Bijker et al., 2012). Interestingly, over two decades ago, a social constructionist analysis of the nursing informatics literature examined how social factors and contexts influence the development and understanding of nursing informatics. The authors argued that access, competence, and culture inform the use of information technology as a tool for achieving practical and efficient outcomes in nursing. This analysis challenges the dominant narrative of instrumental rationality, advocating for a political epistemology that values the specific contexts of nursing practice (Robinson et al., 1996). In essence, it calls for an understanding of nursing that accounts for the political and social contexts in which nurses work, recognising how these factors influence both practice and knowledge.

The integration and advancement of technology have transformed nursing care, shifting nursing informatics from a technology-centric approach to a more holistic one that incorporates conceptual and role-oriented perspectives. Initially focused on data management and communication, nursing informatics now emphasises the interplay between nurses, data, and care processes. This shift highlights the socio-technical dynamics within nursing informatics, where human, technical, and other influencing actors mutually shape one another. This dynamic has been further impacted by the influx of emerging technologies into nursing care, which increasingly challenge the role of nurses in the face of rapid advancements in artificial intelligence, robotics, digital genetics, haptic technologies, and mixed realities in healthcare.

Digital nursing – navigating contemporary changes in digital technologies within nursing practice

Digital nursing focuses on the integration and utilisation of digital technologies by nurses in their daily practice to enhance patient care and improve operational efficiency (Havard et al., 2024). A systematic review by Krick and colleagues identifies a variety of digital technologies used in nursing, including ICT, robotics, sensors, multiple technologies, electronic health records (EHR), monitoring systems, assistive devices, e-learning, health information systems (HIS), educational technologies, ambient assisted living (AAL), decision support systems, virtual reality, tracking tools, serious games, and patient medical records (PMR) (Krick et al., 2019). Additionally, a taxonomy of digital health concepts now includes extended reality (XR), artificial intelligence (AI), and e-prescribing, offering deeper insight into the challenges and benefits of these technologies for nursing practice (Vasilica et al., 2023). Some of these concepts, and their impact on nursing practice, are briefly discussed below and further elaborated on throughout this book.

Social and digital media have driven an increased reliance on mobile devices, the internet, and social platforms for health information and support. These have become powerful tools for nurses to influence population health by addressing information needs (Vasilica, 2015; Vasilica et al., 2020, 2021), encouraging changes in health-related behaviours (Laranjo et al., 2014; Yang, 2017), and promoting self-management (Merolli et al., 2013; Vasilica et al., 2020). However, despite the demonstrated benefits, clinicians often underestimate the role of social media and question patients' ability to critically evaluate the information they consume (Gamor et al., 2023; Dudina & Judina, 2023). This lack of trust is exacerbated by the widespread dissemination of misinformation and disinformation in digital spaces. Misinformation, combined with growing public distrust of science and increased reliance on alternative medicine, can lead to poor health decisions, resulting in harmful outcomes and risks to public safety (Resnick, 2018; Johnson et al., 2021).

Mobile devices, particularly smartphones and health applications, enable nurses to provide remote advice in the digital spaces that people frequently use, such as social media, or through bespoke applications like self-management apps. Smartphones are expected to drive a 'mobile health revolution' due to their accessibility, portability, and increasing affordability (Lucivero & Jongsma, 2018). Mobile health has been incorporated into clinical practice through wearables, apps, and messaging systems, offering wellness programmes and tools for patients with chronic conditions to manage their health independently. These technologies hold great potential in preventing, monitoring, and managing health conditions, particularly in settings where camera technology can play a critical role (Vasilica et al., 2023). To maximise the benefits of mobile health, nurse professionals must deepen their understanding of these complex interactions to effectively support patients in making informed medical decisions (Patrick et al., 2022).

Telehealth offers agile solutions for the delivery and management of healthcare services directly to individuals in their homes or for remote care provided by healthcare professionals via digital platforms (Blandford et al., 2020). The technologies that support telehealth are rapidly expanding and include wearable devices, smartphones, and smart home systems. Smart homes can be equipped with environmental and personal sensors, connected through the Internet of Things (IoT), allowing for continuous monitoring of patient health. During the COVID-19 pandemic, telehealth became one of the most prominent and rapidly expanded strategies for healthcare delivery (Joo, 2022). Nurses are now able to provide personalised care on demand via the internet, prompting nursing professionals to rethink how they interact with and care for patients in a remote setting (Wu, 2021).

Wearable devices, such as fitness trackers and smartwatches, monitor health metrics like heart rate, activity levels, and sleep patterns, often integrating with health apps. Medical wearable devices have emerged as one of the most promising areas of technological advancement. These smart devices not only help individuals maintain healthier lifestyles but also continuously collect health data, assisting in disease diagnosis and treatment by tracking physiological parameters and metabolic status (Lu et al., 2020). This technology provides nurses with valuable data, enabling them to monitor vital signs, neurological disorders, diabetes, wound care, maternal and infant health, cardiac conditions, and more (Pannase et al., 2022).

Artificial intelligence (AI) and robotic systems, although still in their infancy, offer promising solutions for nursing care. AI capabilities include machine learning (ML), natural language processing (NLP), behavioural pattern recognition, search engine functionalities, image and sound analysis, environmental perception, databases, information classification, and artificial neural networks. Robotic process automation (RPA) is another critical aspect of AI, involving software robots that automate repetitive tasks, as well as physical robots programmed to perform tasks in real-world settings (Martinez-Ortigosa et al., 2023). AI-powered chatbots and robots are increasingly becoming emotionally responsive, and their potential to support nursing tasks – such as assisting with ambulation, measuring vital signs, administering medications, and adhering to infection control protocols – is actively being explored. Current research highlights AI's use in nursing for patient risk identification, health assessments, patient classification, improved care delivery, medical record management, and workflow optimisation (Martinez-Ortigosa et al., 2023; Ruksakulpiwat et al., 2024). However, AI is not viewed as a complete substitute for the irreplaceable role of medical professionals but rather as a complementary tool (Altamimi et al., 2023). As AI capabilities continue to improve, its role in nursing will need ongoing reassessment, with its uses and potential explored in more detail later in this book.

Digital genomics represents a convergence of genomics and digital medicine, combining the study of genomes with advanced digital technologies. This intersection enables vast amounts of genetic data to be analysed and interpreted through computational methods, machine learning, and artificial intelligence. By integrating these fields, digital genomics facilitates personalised medicine, allowing treatments and preventive measures to be tailored to an individual's genetic profile. Additionally, it enhances the understanding of genetic diseases, supports the development of new therapies, and improves diagnostic accuracy (Bombard et al., 2022).

Blockchain technologies, initially popularised as the foundation of Bitcoin, have expanded beyond financial transactions into numerous fields, including healthcare. In the context of Bitcoin, blockchain allowed people to exchange electronic coins directly within a network without the need for a central authority, such as a bank. Traditional transactions require a trusted third party (TTP), like a bank, which can fail, be hacked, or cause delays and incur additional fees. This reliance creates vulnerabilities due to a single point of failure. Blockchain technologies, like Bitcoin, were developed to eliminate the need for a TTP in electronic transactions. In healthcare, blockchain can have a variety of applications, including managing electronic medical records, overseeing pharmaceutical supply chains, supporting biomedical research and education, enabling remote patient monitoring, and enhancing health data analytics, among other uses (Agbo et al., 2019; Saeed et al., 2022).

Digital health citizenship

One of the most significant challenges in the digital transformation of healthcare is the imbalance regarding who benefits from these advances and how. As we progress, vast aspects of human experience are being transformed into an inexhaustible resource, continuously extracted as data and converted into knowledge. However, this system only thrives if citizens, patients, and clinicians engage with it – by providing data, interacting regularly, and supporting its sustainability. In the near future, it is anticipated that many healthcare interactions will be guided by algorithms and automated features. This shift demands proactive steps to empower communities and encourage public participation in health and well-being, all under the guidance of healthcare professionals, including nurses.

Digital health citizenship is defined as a combination of discourses, technologies, and practices (Petrakaki et al., 2021). It exists at the intersection of biosociality and technosociality. Biosociality refers to social relations formed around biological or pathological factors, while technosociality pertains to social relationships shaped by technology. Petrakaki and colleagues argue that digital technology not only facilitates biological citizenship but also creates new forms of digital health citizenship. These forms include altruistic behaviours related to health data production, fostering a sense of community belonging, and advocating for changes in healthcare services (Petrakaki et al., 2021). While the concept of digital health citizenship offers exciting possibilities for more engaged and informed patients, it also raises important ethical and practical questions about accessibility and equity in care. Nurses, as key facilitators of digital health, are uniquely positioned to help bridge these gaps, ensuring that the benefits of digital tools are accessible to all, not just the digitally literate or technologically privileged.

The transformative effects of digital technology on health citizenship are becoming increasingly evident, particularly in developed healthcare systems. For instance, the UK National Information Board's Personal Health and Care 2020 framework aimed to create 'a technology and data-enabled care system with the citizen at its centre' (2014, p.16). This framework uses terms like 'patients, service users, citizens, and professionals' (National Information Board, 2014, p.7), demonstrating how policies increasingly blur the line between patients and citizens. Moreover, the framework presents technology as a key solution to existing healthcare challenges. Fundamental to the evolution of digital health citizenship is the active participation of patients in generating health data. The concepts of patient activation and engagement are now tightly interwoven with strategies to promote health citizenship, encouraging patients to take a proactive role in their healthcare (Petrakaki et al., 2021).

The broad conceptualisation of engagement encompasses four main dimensions: behavioural, psychological, multidimensional, and social. These dimensions are applied across various fields such as organisational behaviour, education, informatics, psychology, sociology, management, health communication, and political science (Javornik & Mandelli, 2013, p.2). Behavioural studies focus on actions that occur in response to motivational factors (Van Doorn et al., 2010), which, in the context of social media, often involve varying levels of participation in creating and sharing content. Psychological studies, meanwhile, identify emotional and cognitive processes as the primary drivers of behaviour (Javornik & Mandelli, 2013, p.7). This suggests that the multidimensional aspect of engagement involves both behavioural and psychological changes stemming from user experiences with a particular medium.

The social dimension, a complex concept, is concerned with interactions among individuals within a community, as well as between individuals and their environment (Javornik & Mandelli, 2013). This social dimension is further explored by Vasilica (2015), who expanded upon O'Brien and Toms (2008) engagement theory. Vasilica's extended model (2015) **reinforces** that engagement begins with a goal. Following this initial engagement point, factors such as usability, challenge, attention, novelty, interactivity, interaction, and sociability influence ongoing engagement. Other factors – such as time, age, health literacy, information quality, and confidentiality – can also impact continuous engagement. Disengagement, **conversely**, is often driven by environmental factors, health issues, and negativity, though sociability and the quality of shared information can persuade patients to stay engaged (Vasilica, 2015).

Several key factors contribute to the development and strengthening of digital health citizenship, including digital capabilities, health literacy, accessibility, and policies that protect individuals' rights while promoting the ethical use of health data. Digital capabilities (e.g., technical competencies, information and data literacy, communication, collaboration, safety, and problem-solving) are fundamental for navigating the complexities of the digital world, whether for personal, educational, health, or professional purposes. These capabilities are essential not only for patients but also for nurses, who must support patients, carers, and the general public in navigating digital healthcare tools (Mbeah & Vasilica, 2024).

Nursing professionals play a crucial role in promoting digital health citizenship, ensuring that patients are engaged, informed, and empowered throughout their healthcare journeys. Nurses, often the primary point of contact for patients, engage in remote care and coordinate services among various healthcare professionals. In this capacity, nurses can educate and support patients and the public on health issues, preventive measures, and healthy living practices.

To illustrate the transformative effect of digital technologies on nursing practice and education, the following section presents two fictional vignettes. These examples demonstrate the potential benefits and challenges of integrating digital systems into healthcare.

Vignette 2.1 highlights the advantages of using interoperable Electronic Health Records (EHR) to facilitate communication among healthcare professionals.

Vignette 2.1 – From paper-based to interoperable EHR

This vignette highlights the advantages of using interoperable Electronic Health Records (EHR) to facilitate communication among healthcare professionals.

Andy, a patient, arrives at the surgical outpatient department of a multi-specialty hospital for a routine appointment. Helen, an Advanced Nurse Practitioner (ANP), begins Andy's physical examination and notices a surgical scar on his abdomen. When questioned, Andy mentions he had surgery 30 years ago but cannot recall the details and has no next of kin who could provide further information.

Helen searches Andy's medical folder but finds no relevant details about the surgery. She contacts the hospital's medical records department, which informs her that retrieving old paper-based records will require a formal request and could take up to two weeks. Helen submits the request and schedules a follow-up appointment for Andy six weeks later.

At the follow-up appointment, Helen receives seven folders containing Andy's old records. Unfortunately, the documents are faded, and some are illegible, providing no useful information. In a further attempt to obtain his records, Helen contacts another hospital where Andy received prior treatment, but the EHR systems between the two hospitals are not interoperable. As a result, she is unable to access the records electronically, forcing her to rely on the slow and cumbersome process of requesting physical copies.

Helen's experience underscores the inefficiencies of both paper-based and non-interoperable medical records, illustrating the communication barriers these systems can create among healthcare professionals. Effective communication is critical to delivering high-quality clinical care and reducing medical errors. Fully interoperable EHR systems can mitigate these issues by enabling seamless access to patient records. Healthcare professionals could instantly view relevant patient information such as allergies, medications, lab results, care plans, and referrals, significantly reducing delays in patient care. This vignette emphasises the importance of modernising and integrating medical record systems to improve communication and prevent errors.

Vignette 2.2 – Supporting John, a patient with a motor disability

This vignette demonstrates how digital health technologies, when made accessible, can empower patients with disabilities to take a more active role in managing their health.

John has multiple sclerosis (MS), which impairs his motor functions. Recently diagnosed with diabetes, John is eager to use a self-management app to monitor his blood glucose levels, track his diet, and manage his medications. Nurse Kyle has been assigned to help John access and effectively use the app.

Kyle takes a person-centred approach, starting by asking John about his digital skills and the support he might need, even though John hasn't explicitly mentioned any challenges. Kyle explains that understanding these barriers will enable him to offer appropriate support.

To better assess John's needs, Kyle asks about the digital technology John already uses, how confident he feels with it, and what concerns he has. John explains that while he uses a smartphone for basic tasks and participates in a Facebook group for people with MS, he struggles with apps that require precise touch control due to his motor impairments.

Kyle involves John in the decision-making process, allowing him to choose how he wa nts to be supported. They explore assistive technologies that could help, such as voice-activated commands and stylus pens designed for people with limited motor function. Kyle also considers John's broader digital needs, not just for managing diabetes, but for other aspects of daily life. He suggests apps that could assist with tasks like setting reminders and paying for parking.

Together, Kyle and John create a tailored plan that includes step-by-step guidance on using the app, training sessions for assistive technologies, and support channels for any future digital challenges. Kyle helps John set up the app and demonstrates how to use voice commands for easier navigation. With Kyle's support, John becomes proficient in using the self-management app, which empowers him to better manage his diabetes.

In addition to supporting John's technical needs, Kyle connects him with a support group for people with MS and schedules follow-up sessions to ensure John remains comfortable using the app. He also encourages John to provide feedback so that any necessary adjustments can be made.

The two vignettes illustrate both the benefits and challenges of integrating digital technologies into nursing practice. They highlight how digital transformation requires not only technical tools but also adjustments in broader socio-technical systems including workflows, training, and organisational structures.

Helen's struggle with non-interoperable EHR systems underscores the socio-technical challenges discussed earlier in the chapter. While EHRs offer the potential to streamline care and reduce errors, their effectiveness is hindered by fragmented implementation. This scenario demonstrates that digital tools must be supported by organisational alignment, adequate training, and interoperable systems to truly improve patient outcomes (Lau et al., 2010; Neame et al., 2020).

Furthermore, this vignette highlights the ethical implications of delayed access to patient records, which can compromise care quality. It reinforces the need for modernising medical record-keeping and ensuring that nurses are trained to adapt to these changes (Staggers, 2002).

John's experience illustrates the role of digital tools in promoting patient empowerment and digital health citizenship. By personalising the use of assistive technologies, Kyle ensures that John can actively manage his diabetes despite his motor disability. This aligns with the concept of digital inclusion, emphasising that accessibility is key to equitable healthcare (Petrakaki et al., 2021). This issue is explored in greater depth in Chapter 3.

Nurses, like Kyle, serve as crucial facilitators of digital health, bridging the gap between technology and patient care. This vignette demonstrates how a person-centred approach can empower patients and promote greater independence, showcasing the importance of tailoring digital solutions to individual needs.

Shaping the future of digital nursing, STS perspectives

The integration of technology in healthcare has been ongoing for decades, but the latest advancements necessitate a more immediate transformation of nursing practice into a digitally enabled profession equipped to address complex global healthcare challenges. This calls for a proactive approach from nursing leaders to incorporate digital and technological advancements into both health and social care education and practice.

Science and Technology Studies (STS) provide a framework for understanding the intricate nature of technological implementation, illustrating that it extends beyond mere technical tools. STS highlights the importance of specific contexts and environments in shaping nursing practice and knowledge application. Within digital nursing, work systems consist of interdependent technical and social subsystems that must be jointly optimised for maximum performance. This requires an emphasis on the interaction between social, technical, and even environmental components, rather than isolating their individual properties. For instance, the

TABLE 2.1 Examples of STS dimensions applied to digital nursing practice

STS Dimension	*Nursing Practice*
Technical	*Physical systems*: Technology, hardware, software, facilities *Software*: EHR (e.g., NHS England accredited systems like Allscripts, Cerner, DXC, IMS Maxims, Nervecentre, Meditech, TPP, System C), chatbots, digital genetics, apps *Hardware*: Mobile devices, telehealth devices, medical equipment, internet connections, robots, sensors, assistive devices *Human-computer interface*: Simple designs, minimal clicks, interoperability
Processes/ procedures	Clinical content, tasks/goals, influencing factors, connectivity
Social	*People*: Nurses *Culture*: Team dynamics and professional norms *Structure*: Organisational structures at macro/meso levels – nursing teams, informatics, leadership, digital health citizens, IT teams *Environment*: Workflow, communication processes, organisational policies

adoption of electronic health records (EHRs) involves more than just technical training – it requires modifications in workflow, communication patterns, and the culture of the healthcare institution. Table 2.1 (below) provides examples of how these STS dimensions apply to digital nursing practice.

Digitally enabled care and the joy of practice

Digitally enabled care is increasingly seen as a powerful mechanism for restoring the "joy of practice" to nursing (Phillips et al., 2024). The rapid pace of technological innovation has expanded the scope of nursing, offering tools that support care delivery while enhancing operational efficiency. However, the integration of these tools brings challenges that extend beyond technical know-how, requiring nurses to balance the technological and human elements of care.

One of the key issues explored earlier in this chapter is the co-construction of digital technologies and nursing practices (Bijker et al., 2012). The relationship between nurses and the tools they use is not static; nurses are actively involved in shaping how digital technologies are implemented, adapted, and refined within the clinical context. For example, electronic health records (EHRs) offer nurses the ability to access patient information more efficiently, but this benefit can only be fully realised when accompanied by appropriate training, workflow adaptation, and cultural shifts within healthcare organisations. If these socio-technical systems are not optimised, nurses may experience frustration, burnout, and a loss of job satisfaction rather than the "joy of practice" that technology promises.

The importance of a holistic perspective

As discussed earlier, the implementation of technologies such as telehealth, AI, and wearable devices transforms nursing roles. These tools enable nurses to offer remote support, monitor patient health in real-time, and use data-driven insights to make more informed decisions (Vasilica et al., 2023). However, these innovations also raise new ethical and professional challenges. Nurses must navigate the fine line between technological reliance and maintaining the human element of care, especially when dealing with vulnerable populations such as patients with disabilities (illustrated in Vignette 2.2). As technology becomes more integrated into care, nurses must ensure that the use of digital tools does not unintentionally widen health disparities or alienate patients who may struggle with digital and health literacy (Krick et al., 2019).

In this context, an STS approach allows us to evaluate these complexities by highlighting the interplay between the technical, social, and environmental dimensions of nursing practice (Bijker et al., 2012). The example of AI discussed earlier in this chapter illustrates how this interplay can shape nursing practice. AI tools offer promising capabilities in areas such as patient risk identification and workflow optimisation (Martinez-Ortigosa et al., 2023). However, nurses must also contend with the non-human actors, such as algorithms, that are becoming increasingly embedded in care processes. These tools may alter decision-making processes, prompting nurses to develop new competencies to critically evaluate AI-generated insights while maintaining their professional autonomy (Altamimi et al., 2023).

Reassessing nursing theories in the digital age

One of the critical insights offered by the STS framework is its focus on the socio-technical nature of digital nursing. Traditional nursing theories often emphasise the human aspects of care, compassion, clinical decision-making, and patient-centredness, while overlooking how digital tools mediate and shape these processes (Wynn & Garwood-Cross, 2024). In contrast, an STS perspective recognises that technology is not a neutral tool; it is an active participant in care delivery. For example, EHR systems, telehealth platforms, and wearable devices create new dynamics in nurse-patient relationships, communication flows, and care processes.

Nursing can be viewed as a dynamic practice shaped by an ever-evolving network of human and non-human actors (Wickramasinghe et al., 2007). These actors mutually influence each other, as seen in the earlier vignettes. For example, in Vignette 1.1, the non-interoperable EHR systems hinder effective communication between healthcare professionals, directly impacting the nurse's ability to provide timely and accurate care. By considering technology as an agent within the care environment, the STS framework allows for a deeper exploration of how nursing practice can adapt to ensure that these systems complement, rather than complicate, patient care.

Chapter summary

Looking ahead, digital technologies such as AI, robotics, and blockchain will continue to push the boundaries of what is possible in nursing practice. The chapter has explored how these technologies offer exciting possibilities but also bring new responsibilities for nurses. For instance, AI-powered systems can assist in diagnosis and treatment recommendations, but nurses must remain vigilant about the ethical implications of relying on algorithmic decision-making, especially when it comes to issues such as data privacy, bias, and transparency. Similarly, while blockchain technology promises to enhance the security of health data, nurses will need to develop new competencies in data management and digital ethics to protect patient privacy in increasingly complex digital ecosystems.

The STS perspective encourages nursing leaders to adopt a proactive, interdisciplinary approach to integrating digital innovations into nursing practice. It challenges nurses not just to be passive recipients of technology but to actively shape and influence the development of digital tools. By engaging with policymakers, technology developers, and patients, nurses can ensure that these technologies serve the broader goal of improving health outcomes and patient care while preserving the essential human elements of nursing.

References

Agbo, C. C., Mahmoud, Q. H., & Eklund, J. M. (2019). Blockchain technology in healthcare: A systematic review. *Healthcare, 7*(2), 56. https://doi.org/10.3390/healthcare7020056

Altamimi, I., Altamimi, A., Alhumimidi, A. S., Altamimi, A., & Temsah, M.-H. (2023). Artificial Intelligence (AI) chatbots in medicine: A supplement, not a substitute. *Cureus.* https://doi.org/10.7759/cureus.40922

Bijker, W. E., Hughes, T. P., & Pinch, T. (2012). *The social construction of technological systems: New directions in the sociology and history of technology.* MIT Press.

Blandford, A., Wesson, J., Amalberti, R., AlHazme, R., & Allwihan, R. (2020). Opportunities and challenges for telehealth within, and beyond, a pandemic. *The Lancet Global Health, 8*(11). https://doi.org/10.1016/s2214-109x(20)30362-4

Bombard, Y., Ginsburg, G. S., Sturm, A. C., Zhou, A. Y., & Lemke, A. A. (2022). Digital health-enabled genomics: Opportunities and challenges. *The American Journal of Human Genetics, 109*(7), 1190–1198. https://doi.org/10.1016/j.ajhg.2022.05.001

Dowding, D. (2024). Clinical decision support. In N. Phillips, G. Stacey, & D. Dowding (Eds.), *Harnessing digital technology and data for nursing practice* (1st ed., pp. 85–93). Elsevier.

Dudina, V., & Judina, D. (2023). The use of social media in the self-management of chronic diseases: Views of patients and doctors. *European Journal of Public Health, 33*(Supplement_2). https://doi.org/10.1093/eurpub/ckad160.1133

Gamor, N., Dzansi, G., Konlan, K. D., & Abdulai, E. (2023). Exploring social media adoption by nurses for nursing practice in rural Volta, Ghana. *Nursing Open, 10*(7), 4432–4441. https://doi.org/10.1002/nop2.1685

Graves, J. R., & Corcoran-Perry, S. (1996). The study of nursing informatics. *Holistic Nursing Practice, 11*(1), 15–24. https://doi.org/10.1097/00004650-199610000-00005

Hannah, K. J., Ball, M. J., & Edwards, M. J. A. (2006). *Introduction to nursing informatics.* Springer.

Hardey, M. (1999). Doctor in the house: The internet as a source of lay health knowledge and the challenge to expertise. *Sociology of Health & Illness, 21*(6), 820–835. https://doi.org/10.1111/1467-9566.00185

Havard, M., Whistance, M., Johns, G., Drew, S., Cusens, C., Thomas, S., Khalil, S., Ogonovsky, M., & Ahuja, A. (2024). Defining digital nursing. *British Journal of Nursing, 33*(2), 72–77. https://doi.org/10.12968/bjon.2024.33.2.72

Javornik, A., & Mandelli, A. (2013). Research categories in studying customer engagement. In *Proceedings of Academy of Marketing Conference*, Cardiff, UK.

Johnson, S. B., Parsons, M., Dorff, T., Moran, M. S., Ward, J. H., Cohen, S. A., Akerley, W. Bauman, J., Hubbard, J., Spratt, D. E., Bylund, C. L., Swire-Thompson, B., Onega, T., Scherer, L. D., Tward, J., & Fagerlin, A. (2021). Cancer misinformation and harmful information on Facebook and other social media: A brief report. *JNCI: Journal of the National Cancer Institute, 114*(7), 1036–1039. https://doi.org/10.1093/jnci/djab141

Joo, J. Y. (2022). Nurse-led telehealth interventions during COVID-19. *CIN: Computers, Informatics, Nursing, 40*(12), 804–813. https://doi.org/10.1097/cin.0000000000000962

Krick, T., Huter, K., Domhoff, D., Schmidt, A., Rothgang, H., & Wolf-Ostermann, K. (2019). Digital technology and nursing care: A scoping review on acceptance, effectiveness and efficiency studies of informal and formal care technologies. *BMC Health Services Research, 19*(1). https://doi.org/10.1186/s12913-019-4238-3

Laranjo, L., Arguel, A., Neves, A. L., Gallagher, A. M., Kaplan, R., Mortimer, N., Mendes, G. A., & Lau, A. Y. (2014). The influence of social networking sites on health behavior change: A systematic review and meta-analysis. *Journal of the American Medical Informatics Association, 22*(1), 243–256. https://doi.org/10.1136/amiajnl-2014-002841

Lau, F., Kuziemsky, C., Price, M., & Gardner, J. (2010). A review on systematic reviews of health information system studies. *Journal of the American Medical Informatics Association, 17*(6), 637–645. https://doi.org/10.1136/jamia.2010.004838

Lu, L., Zhang, J., Xie, Y., Gao, F., Xu, S., Wu, X., & Ye, Z. (2020). Wearable health devices in health care: Narrative systematic review. *JMIR mHealth and uHealth, 8*(11). https://doi.org/10.2196/18907

Lucivero, F., & Jongsma, K. R. (2018). A mobile revolution for healthcare? Setting the agenda for bioethics. *Journal of Medical Ethics, 44*(10), 685–689. https://doi.org/10.1136/medethics-2017-104741

Martinez-Ortigosa, A., Martinez-Granados, A., Gil-Hernández, E., Rodriguez-Arrastia, M., Ropero-Padilla, C., & Roman, P. (2023). Applications of artificial intelligence in nursing care: A systematic review. *Journal of Nursing Management, 1–12*. https://doi.org/10.1155/2023/3219127

Mbeah, H., & Vasilica, C. M. (2024) Supporting digital literacy. In N. Phillips, D. Dowding & G. Stacey (Eds.), *Harnessing digital technology and data for nursing practice* (1st ed.). Elsevier. 9780443111600.

Merolli, M., Gray, K., & Martin-Sanchez, F. (2013). Health outcomes and related effects of using social media in chronic disease management: A literature review and analysis of affordances. *Journal of Biomedical Informatics, 46*(6), 957–969. https://doi.org/10.1016/j.jbi.2013.04.010

National Information Board. (2014). *Personalised health and care 2020: Using data and technology to transform outcomes for patients and citizens: A framework for action.* Department of Health.

Neame, M. T., Sefton, G., Roberts, M., Harkness, D., Sinha, I. P., & Hawcutt, D. B. (2020). Evaluating health information technologies: A systematic review of framework recommendations. *International Journal of Medical Informatics, 142*, 104247. https://doi.org/10.1016/j.ijmedinf.2020.104247

Nimmagadda, A., Stanley, I., Karliner, J., & Orris, P. (2018). Global substitution of mercury-based medical devices in the sector. In *Water and sanitation-related diseases and the changing environment: Challenges, interventions, and preventive measures* (2nd ed., pp. 189–196). John Wiley & Sons, Inc. https://doi.org/10.1002/9781119415961.ch15

O'Brien, H. L., & Toms, E. G. (2008). What is user engagement? A conceptual framework for defining user engagement with technology. *Journal of the American Society for Information Science and Technology, 59*(6), 938–955. https://doi.org/10.1002/asi.20801

Pannase, K., Mahakalkar, M. M., & Gomase, K. (2022). Benefits of wearable technology to provide efficient nursing care. *Proceedings of the 2022 3rd International Conference on Electronics and Sustainable Communication Systems (ICESC)*, 1084, 24–27. https://doi.org/10.1109/icesc54411.2022.9885590

Patrick, M., Venkatesh, R. D., & Stukus, D. R. (2022). Social media and its impact on health care. *Annals of Allergy, Asthma & Immunology, 128*(2), 139–145. https://doi.org/10.1016/j.anai.2021.09.014

Petrakaki, D., Hilberg, E., & Waring, J. (2021). The cultivation of digital health citizenship. *Social Science & Medicine, 270*, 113675. https://doi.org/10.1016/j.socscimed.2021.113675

Phillips, N., Stacey, G., & Dowding, D. (2024). *Harnessing digital technology and data for nursing practice* (1st ed.). Elsevier.

Pickler, R. H., & Dorsey, S. G. (2021). Shifting paradigms in nursing science. *Nursing Research, 71*(1), 1–2. https://doi.org/10.1097/nnr.0000000000000558

Reid, L., Maeder, A., Button, D., Breaden, K., & Brommeyer, M. (2021). Defining nursing informatics: A narrative review. *Studies in Health Technology and Informatics*. https://doi.org/10.3233/shti210680

Resnick, M. J. (2018). Re: Use of alternative medicine for cancer and its impact on survival. *Journal of Urology, 200*(4), 688–690. https://doi.org/10.1016/j.juro.2018.07.015

Robinson, K., Robinson, H., Davies, H., & Davis, H. (1996). Towards a social constructionist analysis of nursing informatics. *Health Informatics, 2*(4), 179–187. https://doi.org/10.1177/146045829600200402

Ruksakulpiwat, S., Thorngthip, S., Niyomyart, A., Benjasirisan, C., Phianhasin, L., Aldossary, H., Ahmed, B., & Samai, T. (2024). A systematic review of the application of artificial intelligence in nursing care: Where are we, and what's next? *Journal of Multidisciplinary Healthcare, 17*, 1603–1616. https://doi.org/10.2147/jmdh.s459946

Saeed, H., Malik, H., Bashir, U., Ahmad, A., Riaz, S., Ilyas, M., Bukhari, W. A., & Khan, M. I. (2022). Blockchain technology in healthcare: A systematic review. *PLoS One, 17*(4). https://doi.org/10.1371/journal.pone.0266462

Scholes, M., & Barber, B. (1980). Towards nursing informatics. In D. A. D. Lindberg & S. Kaihara (Eds.), *Medinfo 1980* (pp. 70–73). North-Holland.

Schwirian, P. M. (1989). The Ni Pyramid—A model for research in nursing informatics. *Computers and Medicine*, 291–294. https://doi.org/10.1007/978-1-4612-3622-1_29

Sipes, C. (2019). *Nursing informatics: Definition, evolution, guiding principles, expectations*. Springer Publishing.

Staggers, N. (2002). The evolution of definitions for nursing informatics: A critical analysis and revised definition. *Journal of the American Medical Informatics Association, 9*(3), 255–261. https://doi.org/10.1197/jamia.m0946

van Doorn, J., Lemon, K. N., Mittal, V., Nass, S., Pick, D., Pirner, P., & Verhoef, P. C. (2010). Customer engagement behavior: Theoretical foundations and research directions. *Journal of Service Research, 13*(3), 253–266. https://doi.org/10.1177/1094670510375599

Vasilica, C. (2015). *Impact of using social media to increase patient information provision, networking and communication.* United Kingdom: University of Salford. https://salford-repository.worktribe.com/output/1405786/impact-of-using-social-media-to-increase-patient-information-provision-networking-and-communication

Vasilica, C. M., Brettle, A., & Ormandy, P. (2020). A co-designed social media intervention to satisfy information needs and improve outcomes of patients with chronic kidney disease: Longitudinal study. *JMIR Formative Research, 4*(1), e13207–e13207. https://doi.org/10.2196/13207

Vasilica, C., Oates, T., Clausner, C., Ormandy, P., Barratt, J., & Graham-Brown, M. (2021). Identifying information needs of patients with iga nephropathy using an innovative social media–stepped analytical approach. *Kidney International Reports, 6*(5), 1317–1325. https://doi.org/10.1016/j.ekir.2021.02.030

Vasilica, C., & Ormandy, P. (2017). Methods for studying information provision, networking and communication in patient support groups. In C. Urquhart, F. Hamad, D. Tbaishat, & A. Yeoman (Eds.), *Information systems: Process and practice* (pp. 205–233). London: Facet Publishing.

Vasilica, C., Wynn, M., Davis, D., Charnley, K., & Garwood-Cross, L. (2023). The digital future of nursing: Making sense of taxonomies and key concepts. *British Journal of Nursing, 32*(9), 442–446. https://doi.org/10.12968/bjon.2023.32.9.442

Wickramasinghe, N., Bali, R. K., & Tatnall, A. (2007). Using actor network theory to understand network-centric healthcare operations. *International Journal of Electronic Healthcare, 3*(3), 317. https://doi.org/10.1504/ijeh.2007.014551

Winter, A., Ammenwerth, E., Haux, R., Marschollek, M., Steiner, B., & Jahn, F. (2023). *Health information systems: Technological and management perspectives.* Springer Nature.

Wong, P., Brand, G., Dix, S., Choo, D., Foley, P., & Lokmic-Tomkins, Z. (2023). Pre-registration nursing students' perceptions of digital health technology on the future of nursing. *Nurse Educator, 49*(4). https://doi.org/10.1097/nne.0000000000001591

Wu, Y. (2021). Utilization of telehealth and the advancement of nursing informatics during COVID-19 pandemic. *International Journal of Nursing Sciences, 8*(4), 367–369. https://doi.org/10.1016/j.ijnss.2021.09.004

Wynn, M., & Garwood-Cross, L. (2024). Reassembling nursing in the digital age: An actor-network theory perspective. *Nursing Inquiry.* https://doi.org/10.1111/nin.12655

Yang, Q. (2017). Are social networking sites making health behavior change interventions more effective? A meta-analytic review. *Journal of Health Communication, 22*(3), 223–233. https://doi.org/10.1080/10810730.2016.1271065

Zielstorff, R., Abraham, L., Werley, H., Saba, V., & Schwirian, P. (1989). Guidelines for reporting innovations in computer-based information systems for nursing. *Computers in Nursing, 7*(5), 203–208.

3

ETHICAL AND HUMANISTIC DIMENSIONS OF DIGITAL NURSING

*Vanessa Heaslip, Gillian Janes, Marion Waite,
Joanne Reid and Louise Stayt*

Introduction

Many people think that digital health care is a new phenomenon, but in the UK it began in the 1960s when computers were first used in administration, finance and research within the health sector (Kings Fund, 2024). Since then, there has been a growth in all aspects of digital care, with rapid grown most recently driven by the COVID-19 pandemic. This global digital drive within healthcare has been supported by both national and international policy directives (World Health Organisation [WHO], 2022). However, the WHO Global Strategy on Digital Health noted that "digital health will be valued and adopted if it is accessible and supports equitable and universal access to quality health services". They further assert that "digital health should be an integral part of health priorities and benefit people in a way that is ethical, safe, secure, reliable, equitable and sustainable". Both points assert the importance of addressing ethical consideration within the digital space.

Traditionally the focus of ethics in healthcare has largely been centred around Beauchamp and Childress (2001) principles of biomedical ethics: autonomy, beneficence, non-maleficence, and justice. However, Östman et al. (2017) argue for an ontological view of ethics which sees ethics as concerning personal human value, a synthesis of personal values with culture and history. They argue that ethics is fundamentally ethos, the values formed through culture and history and includes a fusion between internal and external perspectives of ethics. In terms of nursing ethics, the International Council of Nurses (ICN) (2021) identify core aspects of ethical nursing practice to be equity and inclusion, promotion of human and cultural rights including the right to choose and the promotion of dignity and respect. These coalesce the values of nursing which include respect, justice, empathy, responsiveness, caring compassion, trustworthiness, and integrity

DOI: 10.4324/9781032714547-3

(ICN, 2021). Central to all these perspectives are the core issues of personhood and what it means to be human, and how this is perceived, enacted, and responded to, all of which is shifting due to the transition to an increasing digital world.

Personhood in the digital age

The digital age continues to shape the digital identities of healthcare consumers and nurses. In turn, the continued development of digital tools and artefacts may enable all parties to act back on the world as humans to shape health services and health service delivery. Of course, these processes are not without challenges, contradictions, and different points of view.

Identity in the digital age

The development of the internet represents a historical turning point, given its now ubiquitous place in all aspects of many people's everyday lives, albeit at different levels of engagement. Ertzscheid (2016) identifies three distinct historical phases that have shaped human digital identity:

1 The Information Age of the Web through the work of Tim Berners-Lee in creating the World Wide Web in 1992
2 World's live web
3 Information in real-time such as blogs, sites and portals; Social Networks known as the World Life Web

Bearing these historical phases in mind, Ertzscheid defines digital identity as:

> Both the collection of traces (writings, audio/video content, forum messages, sign-in details, etc.) that we leave behind us, consciously or unconsciously, as we browse the network and the reflection of this mass of traces as it appears after being 'remixed' by search engines.
>
> *(Ertzscheid, 2016:6)*

This definition assumes that people engage with the world life web and interact at some level by creating content in the form of text, video, or images that are posted and shared with others.

As the World Wide Web is over 30 years old, many people have lived with it all their lives. Millennials (born between 1981 and 1996) are the first to use and interact with mobile social networks and digital media from birth (Granic et al., 2020). Prensky (2001) coined a term 'digital natives' for this millennial generation. These were people with a command of the digital language using computers, video games, and the internet, making them fundamentally different from older generations, or 'digital immigrants', who needed to adapt their lives to digital tools.

Eynon (2020) argues that while it is essential to understand younger people's use of technology, given the complexity and cultural underpinnings of digital technologies, this definition is problematic because it would now be challenging to term everyone born since 1980 as digital natives because this time period encompasses many diverse people in terms of ages and life stages. Yet, Eynon identifies that 'digital natives' still have currency in policymakers' decisions.

As discussed later in the section, assumptions about generational digital identity may be problematic and have implications for nursing practices, including how we perceive the digital identities and personhood of healthcare consumers. However, as Granic et al. (2020) argue, we are at a critical turning point in the digital age because millennials and Gen Z (born between 1997 and 2012) may not experience the online and offline worlds as distinct.

The scholarly definitions of digital identity have yet to encompass human artificial intelligence (AI). AI has featured prominently in media and academic discourse in recent years and presents an apparent tension between the wonders of AI with its algorithms to make unimaginable scientific breakthroughs and the existential threat of AI to humankind. The humanist thinker Stephen Pinker (2018) reminds us that AI is like any other technology. It is developed incrementally, designed with multiple criteria, tested before implementation, consistently reviewed for errors and performance, and re-designed if necessary.

What does identity mean in the digital age (for nurses and health care consumers)

The implications for nurse's identity in the digital age concern confronting the boundaries between personal and professional lives because of the implicit link with reputation and balancing reputations with trust. Social network sites have become spaces where many nurses (and others) present their professional digital identities to enhance their voices and standing in scholarly and professional communities. Furthermore, they extend the notion of digital identity to digital personhood. Boyd et al. (2004), in their digital identity analysis, refer to the human metaphor of the presentation of self. Due to the lack of visual presence in computer-mediated communication (CMC), digital identity and personhood concern performance, and people need to create new ways to present themselves and read the signs of others, which is an embodied interaction. This means that the person makes a user profile, including personal information, based on what the person would like an observant audience to notice. However, the fact that people are traceable and issues concerning security, means that digital identity is difficult to control (Ertzscheid, 2016). Nevertheless, as Ertzscheid argues, digital identities are essential for individuals, which is linked with Maslow's hierarchy of needs (1943): the need for security (use identity), the need for love and belonging (digital communities), and the need for self-esteem through reputation to reach self-actualisation.

Equally, people with enduring health conditions may use social networking sites to present their identities, create social narratives concerning their lived experiences, and aspire to achieve self-actualisation through digital means. It is estimated that 40% of healthcare consumers worldwide use social media for their healthcare needs (Guraya et al., 2021). The implications for digital professional identity mean that people entering the nursing profession have grown up in the digital age, and nurse educators need to understand how undergraduates' digital' life experiences may shape their professional identity development without making assumptions about a digital native generation. Giroux and Moreau (2021) collected the content that undergraduate nurses posted to their social media accounts. Postings concerning advocacy represented the strongest theme and included reactions to media news stories about policy and public health issues such as vaccinations, nursing culture and work, mental health and addiction. Nursing students also posted about nursing identity (some identified as nurses), socialisation and culture, their formal and informal learning experiences and shared educational tools, job opportunities, and relevant resources. However, a liminal space was noted between posts that appeared to convey an emergent understanding of the nursing profession and nursing roles and posts that appeared unprofessional. While social media can be a tool to promote professional identity, there may also be blurred boundaries between professional and unprofessional territories (Guraya et al., 2021). Therefore, it may be more challenging for those raised in a digital age to understand how to navigate the boundaries, yet there is limited evidence of guidance regarding professionalism in the digital era within nursing preparatory programmes (Guraya et al., 2021).

A critical aspect of nurses' professional identity concerns delivery of nursing care in the digital age. This may include technology replacing or being used to assist with nursing tasks, the emergence of technology to support hands-on care, supporting patients with technology to self-manage long-term conditions and nurses' interactions with patients through technology. Knop et al. (2024) identified a lack of studies examining concrete and digital identity-related outcomes for nurses. They undertook a literature review to explore how digital technologies in clinical nursing practice affect nurses' professional identities and identified a delicate balance between technology that enhances nursing care and technology that intrudes into the nursing role. Technology can alter procedures and interactions, but at the same time, it can be co-creating. A critical finding was that nurses taking the lead in digital clinical care experienced positive power relations in their working environments (Knop et al., 2024). They were more likely to transition upwards in the nursing hierarchy, achieving authority and autonomy, leading Knop et al. (2024) to assert that autonomy and authority are prerequisites to shaping technology implementation. For some nurses, however, technology negatively impacted their identity because they experienced a barrier between themselves and the patient because the use of technology shifted the focus of care to patients' objective characteristics.

Consumers' use of social media has been touched upon and the fact that some generations have only lived in the digital age. However, we must be careful when making assumptions about healthcare consumers' digital identities and personhood. This is essential for nurses working with people across the lifespan. Young people's mental health is a frequently featured topic in the media, and for nurses working in young people's services, it is a critical concern. There are many media stories that associate young people's use of technology with mental health issues. Granic et al. (2020) highlight a critical debate concerning young people's (10–24 years) screen time and associations with their mental health. They argue that the notion of screen time is too simplistic. Studies that go beyond counting hours in front of screens are needed. They argue for systematic and objective methods accompanied by a theoretical framework that examines why and how digital media impacts young people and the complex interplay between digital and offline experiences. By combining core principles from clinical, social, and personality psychology with developmental theory, it may be possible to determine the digital experiences that promote healthy normative development as well as emerging serious mental health concerns.

A further health condition that may be associated with digital identities and personhood is diabetes. Diabetes is a long-term condition in which people are encouraged to self-manage supported using technology. Advanced technology such as continuous glucose monitors (CGM) and the artificial pancreas have become available to adults and children with Type 1 diabetes (T1D) in many contexts to replace older methods of measuring blood glucose levels and self-administering insulin. Working in this field of nursing research, the authors have learned how people with diabetes (PWD) make choices about how they use such technology.

CGM is a life-changing technology that reduces the personal burden of managing diabetes and has been long-awaited. However, users' responses to CGM have been mixed (Friedman et al., 2023; Kubiak et al., 2020), with some being considered as not using it to its full potential. There is little understanding of why this is. Waite et al. (2020) found that users needed to develop trust in the technology to provide reliable information about their blood glucose levels. Conversely, adapting to a new self-management technology required an investment of time for learning and potentially intruded on everyday lives because sensors were visible to others, or the device included intrusive alarms signalling critical changes in blood glucose levels. Over time, the adaptations became easier to manage, and users reported an increased understanding and insight into their blood glucose levels, which events required attention and when critical changes were likely to happen. Many users implied that after a period, they were happy to revert to less technological methods of self-monitoring following self-assessment that they had achieved a satisfactory level of learning concerning self-management through temporary use of CGM. This finding is potentially in conflict with bio-medically normative perspectives that people with diabetes (PWD) need to use CGM regularly and indefinitely. This exemplar highlights biomedical dominance of how PWD should self-manage their condition, instead we argue for a person-centred approach to reach a better understanding of how PWD use technology in the context of their everyday lives.

Reflection through the lens of a humanising theoretical framework

Todres et al. (2009) offer a humanising theoretical framework to explore a mutual and productive relationship between health care and qualitative research to inform care. Their definition of humanisation upholds a perspective or places value on what it means to be human and furthermore acts on that concern. The framework provides dimensions expressed along a continuum (Table 3.1); these are not considered to be good or bad but rather provide a humanising lens.

Some of these dimensions are considered below in terms of digitalisation and digital healthcare.

- *Objectification-* Examples of objectification include labelling young people as 'digital natives' or objectifying their screen time duration as a factor in their mental well-being. Objectification may lead to assumptions about young peoples' needs and experiences, overlooking their insider-ness, meaning that their care or the research approaches used to inform it may be inappropriate.
- *Agency/passivity* – The medical model can dominate care delivery. In diabetes, the discovery of insulin by Banting and Best (Pickup, 2015) was a step-change in human science. However, an over concern with objective outcomes such as blood glucose levels runs the risk of rendering the PWD a passive recipient of care and treatment. Many PWD experience multiple challenges in self-managing their diabetes. Some have experienced frustration that innovative technologies are not widely or equitably available. For example, highly motivated and tech-savvy PWD formed the #WeAreNotWaiting movement. Their agency led to them developing a do-it-yourself artificial pancreas which integrates a CGM, insulin pump, and Smartphone technology (Kesavadev et al., 2020). They openly share their algorithms (through social media and open platforms) to help others achieve glycaemic control and improve quality of life. While this has caused alarm for the medical profession owing to lack of regulation, it has enabled the community to inform artificial pancreas design and reclaim personhood to drive their own care.

TABLE 3.1 Humanising theoretical framework (Todres et al., 2009)

Forms of Humanisation	*Forms of Dehumanisation*
Insiderness	Objectification
Agency	Passivity
Uniqueness	Homogenisation
Togetherness	Isolation
Sense-making	Loss of meaning
Personal journey	Loss of personal journey
Sense of place	Dislocation
Embodiment	Reductionist body

- *Uniqueness/homogeneity* – Nurses in the Knop et al. (2024) study identified that technology negatively impacted their identity because they experienced it created a barrier between themselves and the patient because it promoted a shift towards patients' objective characteristics. This means that unique relationships with patients are lost, which may impact on the achievement of person centred, individualised care.
- *Togetherness/isolation* – As discussed earlier the use of social networking sites for nurses and consumers of health care leads to a delicate balance between maintaining privacy while participating in online communities, however they can provide a sense of belonging. Clearly for the participants (undergraduate nurses) in Giroux and Moreau's (2021) study, participation in social media used it to support and demonstrate their formative professional digital identities as nurses.
- *Personal/Loss of personal journey* – Like many other chronic conditions, diabetes is a life-long experience. Yet often studies that examine how technology can support PWD are frequently undertaken outside the person's normal context and often from a biomedical perspective which does not reflect their personal journey of living with diabetes. Yet research which focusses on the wider aspects is important. For example, an examination of how technology devices for adults with Type 1 diabetes are adopted, carried, and used in everyday contexts was done by O'Kane et al. (2015). The research identified that participants reported a wide variety of normalisation of technology use across a continuum of public, personal, and professional usage. For example, in some situations this led to hiding a device, whereas in other situations was confident to show it off.

As these examples illustrate, the humanisation framework is a useful tool for exploring digitalisation and the importance of 'seeing the person' as part of the nursing interaction.

Provision of patient-centred care in digital age

As noted previously, the rapid evolution and introduction of digital health technologies in the last two decades have revolutionised healthcare delivery. Innovations such as care robots, artificial intelligence, clinical decision support tools, electronic health records, telehealth monitoring, and surveillance devices have dramatically impacted nurses, the nature and flow of their work, care delivery, and their interpersonal relationships with those for whom they are caring (Laukka et al., 2023).

Concurrent with the emergence of digital health technologies in the 21st century has been a cultural shift from a disease-centred approach to healthcare delivery towards person-centred care (PCC). This approach values the holistic well-being of patients by integrating their voices, preferences, and needs into every aspect of care (McCormack et al., 2024). Person centred care aims to humanise healthcare provision through active patient involvement and partnership between healthcare professionals, patients, their families, and carers in all decision-making processes, prioritising individual patients' preferences, needs, and values (Leonardsen et al., 2023). A patient-centred approach to care delivery is thought to improve patient satisfaction, lead to better health and reduce hospitalisations as well as having economic benefits (McCormack et al., 2021). Consequently, international bodies such as the World Health Organisation have endorsed PCC as a fundamental aspect of healthcare delivery, promoting policies and practices that prioritise patient engagement and responsiveness (WHO, 2016).

Patient-centred care and digital health technologies have evolved concurrently but often independently, each necessitating a nuanced cultural shift in nurses' roles and the delivery of care. Despite their discrete evolution, there is a natural alignment between PCC and digital innovations. Personal Centred Care highlights the potential of digital tools to empower patients, providing them with information and resources to manage their health and actively engage in healthcare decisions (Leonardsen et al., 2023). Similarly, digital innovations can support the PCC agenda by enhancing patient safety, streamlining care, facilitating decision-making, improving care integration and coordination, and fostering collaboration between patients and healthcare providers (Villa García et al., 2022). However, the relationship between PCC and digital health technologies is not viewed as symbiotic by all. Concerns about digital health technologies have been raised in the research literature, suggesting that their adoption may reduce nurse-patient interactions and communication (Forde-Johnston et al., 2023), reduce compassionate care, detach the nurse from the patient and depersonalise and fragment care (Wharton et al., 2019), widen inequity of health care services (Yao et al., 2022), and present risks to privacy and data protection (Grande et al., 2020).

Despite the apparent dissonance between digital technologies and person-centred care, it is important to remember, as Sandelowski (1998) identifies, that the most enduring image of nursing is Florence Nightingale, the 'lady with the lamp'. Nightingale used the illumination from a candle to assess and monitor her patients, guarding against sickness and deterioration. Today, nurses have a range of advanced devices and digital technologies to help them understand and care for patients. Technologies, in varying degrees of sophistication, have therefore always been integral to nursing and patient care.

Person-centred care overview

Person-centred care is pervasive across healthcare systems and often considered synonymous with good quality health care. It has been widely embraced by healthcare providers the world over and encompasses the individual, right through to the broader care system in which that individual is situated. McCormack et al. (2024) contend that PCC consists of the macro-perspective, which considers systems, organisations and policy, and micro-perspective, which considers individual

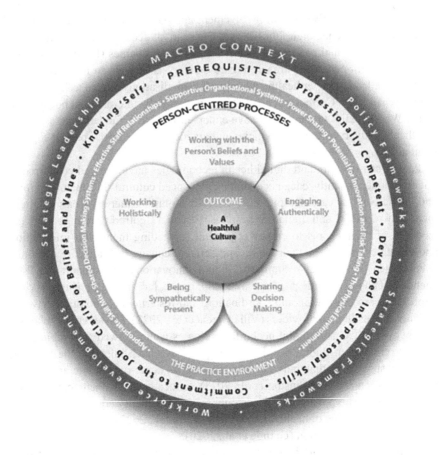

FIGURE 3.1   McCormack and McCance Framework for Person-Centred Care (McCormack et al., 2021).

interactions between, and experiences of service users and providers. This view is consistent with the McCormack and McCance Framework for Person Centred Care (McCormack et al., 2021) (Figure 3.1) which describes a "macro context" concerned with policy and strategic frameworks, workforce developments and strategic leadership; "prerequisites" which focus on the attributes of staff; the "practice environment" which focuses on the context in which healthcare is experienced; and "person-centred processes" which incorporate individualised components of PCC, such as a person's beliefs and values, shared decision-making, holism, and authentic engagement. Digital health technologies exist across the entire system too; the macro-context, prerequisites, practice environment, and person-centred processes will all influence the development, implementation, and adoption of digital health technologies.

Digital health technologies and the macro-context

Strategic leadership

McCormack and McCance (2021) recognise strategic nurse leadership as crucial for achieving PCC, suggesting that a values-based, authentic leadership approach can create a safe working environment where staff feel empowered to enhance care standards and care cultures. Such nurse leaders may also champion, advocate for, and invest in integrating digital technology into daily practice (Heaslip et al., 2024). The rapid development of digital health technologies has transformed clinical nursing work and processes, presenting nurse leaders with the challenge of supporting teams through the digitalisation of healthcare. This includes navigating the associated changes in nursing practice while maintaining an environment where person-centred care can thrive. Moreover, effective leadership during the development and implementation of digital technologies is considered vital for their successful adoption (MacInnes et al., 2023; Krick et al., 2019).

Effective leadership styles in the context of digital health technologies and person-centred care are uncertain, and Laukka et al. (2023) suggest that this lack of understanding about leadership in these constantly evolving contexts means that nurse leaders may be ill prepared for the leadership role. Preparation and support for nurses leading implementation of digital health technologies, certainly seems lacking. Gjellebæk et al. (2020) described how nurse leaders lacked competence in innovation processes and organisational development in the digital context. Sharpp et al. (2019) described this as poor onboarding and education.

Despite the lack of preparation, nurse leaders have significant potential to innovate, develop, and implement digital health technologies within the context of PCC. They are uniquely positioned to understand the prerequisites for PCC that digital technologies can support. Additionally, nurse leaders possess a deep understanding of the populations that these technologies aim to benefit and, crucially, have direct access to these groups. This access facilitates end-user involvement and partnership in technological developments, ensuring that digital solutions remain patient-centred (Laukka et al., 2023). Burgess and Honey (2022) suggest nurse leaders are essential to mediate between digital health implementation priorities and clinical workflow. Moreover, nurse leaders have a comprehensive understanding of the broader macro-context necessary to ensure person-centred care, which is essential for maintaining high-quality and safe patient care. Thus, nursing and midwifery leaders are ideally placed to bridge the clinical-technical divide yet their leadership voice in digital health is largely missing, and at best hidden (Janes et al., 2024).

Heaslip et al. (2024) recognised the potential for nurse leadership of digital health innovations at all levels of healthcare delivery from senior nurses leading strategic framework and policy development, to nurses at the point of care delivery who may bridge the gap between patient care and the digital technologies that enhance it. Nurses at the point of care delivery, not only administer direct patient care but also play an essential role in the digital optimisation of healthcare processes, improving patient outcomes using technology (Heaslip et al., 2024). Burgess and Honey (2022) highlight the nurse leader as an advocate to ensure the nurse voice is heard during the development and integration of digital technologies. Digital leaders across the whole landscape of PCC from person-centred processes through to the macro-context are fundamental to the successful development and integration of digital technologies and PCC. The challenge to the nursing community is therefore to grow and develop nurse leaders who may authentically lead PCC, who also have agency, capability, and capacity to strategically lead digital innovation, implementation, and adoption of digital health technologies.

Safety and governance

Hesitancy in adopting novel digital technologies is often attributed to a lack of confidence in privacy and data security (MacInnes et al., 2021; Sheikh et al., 2021). Cybersecurity and privacy concerns erode trust among patients and healthcare providers, reinforcing health systems' reluctance to share data (Abernethy et al., 2022). However, robust mechanisms for storing, accessing, and sharing health information and patient data are fundamental to person-centred care (PCC). Key hallmarks of PCC, such as shared decision-making, integrated, and continuous care, rely on secure but accessible information and data.

Cybersecurity and privacy concerns are well-founded. Tin et al. (2023) highlighted that cyberattacks and healthcare breaches are among the most costly and disruptive issues facing healthcare today, with nearly 300 million people in the US affected by breaches over the last decade. The challenge of adopting digital health technologies within PCC frameworks lies in achieving the correct balance between accessibility and data security. The greater the accessibility of data, the higher the risk to its security. PCC often relies on patients and multi-professional healthcare providers across different organisations accessing patient data and health information. Digital health technologies, such as electronic health records (EHRs), are obvious tools to facilitate this. However, MacInnes et al. (2021) suggest that organisations actively frustrate or restrict the successful adoption of digital health technologies like EHR, through their own policies and procedures. Interorganisational data sharing is often forbidden or made so complicated that it becomes prohibitively expensive or time-consuming. Conversely, Tangari et al. (2021) reported serious privacy concerns and inconsistent privacy practices associated with widely accessible mobile health applications, warning clinicians to exercise caution when recommending their use to patients. This imbalance between security and accessibility reflects a misalignment in data governance policies and frameworks within and between organisations that can hamper seamless PCC.

MacInnes et al. (2021) and Keshta and Odeh (2021) suggest little is being done in terms of developing evidence-based strategies and policies to manage cyberthreats and privacy concerns with digital health technologies. A challenge facing digital leaders is to develop policies and frameworks that simultaneously address security and privacy concerns while optimising the use of digital health technologies that facilitate and enhance person-centred care.

Digital health technologies, prerequisites, and the practice environment

In terms of prerequisites and the practice environment, there are two main areas; Digital literacy (covered later in the chapter) and time.

Nurses time represents the single highest cost in healthcare therefore enhancing the efficiency and effectiveness of care delivery is a key driver for digital health technology innovation. Technologies are designed to increase nurses' productivity by improving workflows, automating, and standardising processes and improving access to information required for effective and timely clinical decisions. The adoption and assimilation of artificial intelligence-based health technologies such as clinical decision support systems are reported to improve clinical performance and workflows therefore saving time. Bar-code Medication Administration technologies may reduce the time spent conducting the actual task but also, due to the significant reduction of medication errors, save time in the subsequent management of incidents and adverse events (Naidu & Alicia 2019; Owens et al., 2020). Moore et al. (2020) surmises that digital technologies redistribute nurses' time allowing for the delivery of "value-adding" care, such as direct care, and communicating with patients, carers, and other staff.

Conversely, introduction of digital health technologies has been reported to increase the time burden on the nurse. A systematic review by Moore et al. (2020) reported cumbersome systems, duplications of work, distrust of the technologies' capabilities, lack of digital literacy, limitations of the technology requiring "workarounds" and adaptive actions, multi-tasking, and interruptions to workflow due to the demands of technology, as burdens on nurses' time. Kang et al. (2023) participants reported a significantly increased workload associated with the use of socially assistive care robots and suggested that due to the robot's functional limitations, complex programming, and user demands, they felt charged with caring for both the patient and the technology. Taft et al. (2023) assert that digital health technologies' persistent hazards and annoyances distract the nurse from delivering effective patient-centred care causing moral distress and increasing the risk of occupational burnout.

Digital health technologies have the potential to save nurses time, but they can also become burdensome with variable impact PCC. Technologies that actively enhance PCC are a worthwhile investment of nurses' time. Conversely, when the benefits to patient care are less clear, nurses may view them as burdensome. To maximise the potential for PCC, technologies should complement nurses' workflows and activities while providing clear benefits to patients. Balanced consideration of the relative benefits and burdens for all stakeholders is required during the design, implementation, and adoption phases of digital health technology. This can only be achieved through the active engagement of nurses and healthcare consumers from the outset.

Digital health technologies and person-centred processes

Communication and the therapeutic nurse-patient relationship

Engaging authentically in person-centred care requires a commitment to understanding and respecting each patient's unique needs and preferences, fostering open and compassionate communication, building trusting relationships, and creating a supportive and empowering care environment (McCormack et al., 2021). Since the beginning of the digital health revolution, there has been anxiety that the adoption of health technologies might impede the ability to foster trusting relationships and communicate compassionately. Early scholars, such as Barnard and Sandelowski (2001), feared a dehumanisation of nursing care associated with the use of technologies. These fears persist, with Farokhzadian et al. (2020) highlighting the potential for technologies to create a disconnect between patients and providers.

The impact of digital health technologies on communication between nurse and patient has been widely discussed in the research literature. Electronic health records (EHRs), a ubiquitous digital health technology, and its impact on communication and interpersonal relationships have been a particular focus. Using EHR appears to change the quality and nature of communications between the nurse and patient (Forde-Johnson et al., 2023). Communication may be impeded by the logistical set-up of the computer, so the technology acts as a physical barrier between nurse and patient (Alkureishi et al., 2021), or by the clinician typing or looking at the screen during conversation (Burridge et al., 2017). Alkureishi et al. (2021) described the computer as the third party in the nurse-patient relationship with patients competing with the computer for the nurse's attention. The presence of the computer and using EHR also changes the nature and content of the communications between nurses and patients. EHR encourages a clinician-led, task-orientated, checklist-focussed communication leading to a more formulaic approach to communication (Forde-Johnston et al., 2023). With a focus on specific tasks and checklists, the opportunity for natural spontaneous conversations between nurse and patient is less. Suboptimal communication because of digital technology use may subsequently hamper the development of a therapeutic relationship (Rathert et al., 2017; Leonardsen et al., 2023).

While acknowledging the potential of technologies to impede authentic engagement, there is evidence that digital health technologies actively enhance communication and engagement. A literature review (Walthall et al., 2022) identified that remote reviews may enhance therapeutic relationships as patients reported feeling they had the undivided attention of the clinicians and were less rushed compared to being reviewed in a busy clinical environment. Clinicians also reported that patients seemed more receptive when consultations were conducted remotely. The use of digital technologies may also enhance authentic engagement by enabling a convenient and timely exchange of information and supporting collaboration between patients, carers, and the multi-disciplinary team (Burkoski et al., 2019; Koltsida & Jonasson, 2021).

A scoping review (Ali et al., 2022) highlighted that compassionate nursing care in relation to the use of digital health technology is continuously evolving; yet how nurses convey compassion and caring behaviours when providing care while using digital health technologies is not well articulated within the research literature. Despite this, nurses are frequently identified as the face and voice of technological innovations (Ali et al., 2022). Nurses, provide digital education to patients and carers, coordinate digital systems, troubleshoot digital health technologies, are often the ones on a video call, and frequently serve as the first point of contact for technology end-users. This uniquely positions nurses to mitigate the potential negative impact of technology on communication and therapeutic relationships while optimising its enhancing effects on authentic engagement.

Shared decision-making

Shared decision-making is at the heart of PCC. Digital health technologies may play a crucial role in the enactment of shared decision-making and therefore PCC. Technologies can improve access to information, enhance communication, act as decision aids, enhance patient engagement, and offer support systems for patients and healthcare providers.

To actively participate in a shared decision all parties require access to accurate and up-to-date information. Digital technologies provide unprecedented access to health information (MacInnes et al., 2021). Patients may select and engage with digital tools and resources such as patient portals, mobile health apps, self-help programmes, monitoring, and tracking data and be more informed and empowered to personalise their health and wellness in accordance with their individual needs, values, and goals (Burkoski et al., 2019). Similarly, healthcare providers may use digital platforms to access and share latest research, evidence-based guidelines and comprehensive patient medical history, treatments and outcomes providing a better understanding of the patients' overall health status (Anderson et al., 2024). Digital platforms may support the integration and consolidation of health information and patient data from various sources and offer potential for shared access to patient data and information. This supports shared decision-making and has been found to lead to better care coordination, decision support and reduce the duplication of interventions and tests (Villa García et al., 2022). However, frequently system incompatibilities lead to data silos where not all the essential information relevant to the patient is recorded or accessible across different platforms and settings (Anderson et al., 2024). This is a widespread and so far, intractable challenge that needs to be addressed (Janes et al, 2024).

Sophisticated data analytics and artificial intelligence (AI) can be used to identify patterns and trends in a patient's health, enabling proactive and preventive care measures individualised to patients risks and needs (Yelne et al., 2023). AI enables large and complex datasets and patient-specific information including genetic data medical history and real-time health metrics which may be used to tailor individualised health plans and care (Johnson et al., 2021). Such tools may support patients' decision-making processes and support consideration of their personal values and preferences leading to targeted and efficient care, improving patient outcomes and satisfaction. However, the effectiveness of any datasets is premised on the quality of inputted information, and this includes capturing data of those who are marginalised and socially excluded. For example, the NHS data dictionary uses the ethnic categories defined in the 2001 census and as such does not include Gypsy, Roma, Travelers as separate ethnic categories but rather subsumes these into the White any other background category (NHS England, 2024) as such the quality of information collated about these communities is poor. So, while the promise of AI in PCC is great, as an emerging technology, the extent to which it supports and improves clinical decision-making remains uncertain. Zhang et al. (2024) highlights that AI clinical decision support systems both enables and constrains decision-making. This can create dilemmas for nurses when the AI-recommended treatment or care plan is incongruent with their own assessment, leading to tinkering with the system or overruling AI-generated decisions (Zhang et al., 2024).

Digital technologies may enhance patient engagement with health behaviours. Health trackers and wearable devices may enable patients to track health metrics such as heart rate, blood pressure, activity levels, glucose levels, which can be shared with healthcare providers to inform shared decision-making (Lu et al., 2020). Digital health technologies may offer alternative sources of support for patients with health conditions. Virtual support groups such as online forums and support groups provide patients with a platform to share experiences and advice, which can inform their decisions and provide emotional support. AI-driven chatbots can answer patient queries and provide information, ensuring that patients have the knowledge they need to participate in decision-making.

Digital health technologies have the potential to significantly enhance shared decision-making by providing patients and healthcare providers with better access to information, improved communication tools, and personalised decision aids. However, challenges such as digital literacy, privacy concerns, and the need for adequate training and system integration must be addressed to fully realise the benefits. By overcoming these challenges, digital health technologies can support more informed, engaged, and empowered patients, leading to better health outcomes and a more collaborative healthcare experience.

Digital exclusion

As noted previously digital health technologies have the potential to improve health outcomes, however this can only be achieved if the technology is safe, fit for purpose, and universally accessible (Heaslip et al., 2024). Yet a recent review by the World Health Organisation European Region (2023) identified that across its' member states (n=53) only just over half have implemented a digital inclusion plan, highlighting a lack of focus on this issue at national policy levels. While there is currently no universally accepted definition of digital exclusion it typically refers to groups and communities unable to use the internet in ways that are needed to fully participate in society (House of Lords, 2023). Within digital exclusion there are issues related to digital infrastructure, access to digital technology, confidence, and digital literacy, none of which can be assumed universally.

Digital access and infrastructure

In terms of infrastructure across Europe, there is not universal coverage. The European Commission (2024) recently identifies limited fibre coverage across Europe (56% of all households and 41% of households in rural areas). In the UK, availability of internet coverage is also a challenge as around 80,000 premises do not have a decent broadband service (House of Lords, 2023). Furthermore, there are also 'not-spots' where no 4G signal is available as these are often located in rural areas as well as deprived urban areas (House of Lords, 2023). In terms of digital infrastructure, there is a recognition that some areas are identified as 'hard to reach'. The Department for Science Innovation and Technology (2023) define these as places which are:

- physically isolated;
- located in areas with neighbours at a considerable distance;
- island locations;
- located in areas where the distance between premises and accessible points of interconnection is substantial;
- in mountain ranges, valleys, marshlands, bogs; and
- areas where there are access-related issues.

The term 'hard to reach' has also previously been used to refer to people (especially those who are socially excluded). It is important however to recognise that geographically, places (such as those noted above) can be hard to reach in terms of digital infrastructure however this is not a term that should be applied to people as their access to digital infrastructure can be hampered by structural and other barriers beyond their control leading them to be underserved. For example, in the UK there are around 1.7 million households that do not have internet access via a mobile phone or broadband internet at home (Office for National Statistics [ONS], 2019). Furthermore, there are around 5.3 million adults (10% of the adult population) who are defined as non-internet users, who have either never used the internet or not used it in the last three months (ONS, 2019). Exploring this further in the UK, there is a north south divide in that there are more people who are non-internet users in the north compared to the south of England (ONS, 2019). Symbiotically people living in the north of the UK are also more likely to experience social exclusion (Dykxhoorn et al., 2024) and have the lowest incomes (ONS, 2021), highlighting the link between digital exclusion, poverty and social exclusion. To address this, there are social tariffs, which typically cost £12–20 per month for people in receipt of social benefits. While these are cheaper than normal tariffs (around £30 per month), in April 2023 only 5.1% of eligible customers (in the UK) had signed up (House of Lords, 2023), highlighting that for many people these cheaper tariffs are outside of their price range. Access to the internet in lower income household can also fluctuate. For example, the recent cost of living crisis in the UK resulted in around 1 million households reducing or cancelling their internet packages (ONS, 2019).

Even if people have the digital infrastructure in terms of internet provision both to and within their home, many do not have the suitable devices to enable internet use. This was highlighted during the COVID-19 national lockdowns when many children and young people struggled to access online classrooms and others struggled to access healthcare support; though since this pandemic device donation schemes run through councils and charities such as the Good Foundation National Device Bank have developed.

Digital literacy

Even if people have access to devices and the internet, they need the confidence and skills to use them. As such, digital literacy/technological competence is fundamental to effective integration of digital health technologies into person-centred or humanised care (Brown et al., 2020; Gaughan et al., 2022).

Population

In the UK around 2.4 million people are unable to complete the single basic task of getting online and over 5 million employed adults cannot complete essential digital work tasks. There are five basic digital skills (Figure 3.2) identified by the Tech Partnership (2018) that can be used to measure digital inclusion.

These five basic skills include the ability to create something from new or complete an online application, search for information on the internet, use the internet to communicate (via email), to purchase things online and have fundamental problem-solving skills such as accessing help online. In 2018 the Digital Tech Partnership identified that 11.3 million people in the UK did not have these five basic skills (Tech Partnership, 2018). Furthermore by 2030 the Office for National Statistics (2019) estimates that basic digital skills are set to become the UK largest skills gap.

Nursing workforce

Research indicates that nurses seldom receive formal education and support to develop digital literacy and are often self-taught. Moreover, nurses report a lack

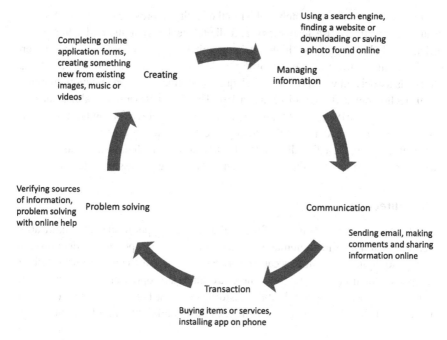

FIGURE 3.2 Five basic digital skills.

Source: Adapted from the Tech Partnership (2018).

of professional development opportunities to enhance their digital skills (Brown et al., 2020; Laukka et al., 2023; Bimerew & Chipps 2022). Consequently, the level of digital literacy varies among the nursing workforce at all levels of seniority (Caton et al., 2024; Isidori et al., 2022).

Digital literacy is often assumed, particularly among younger generations of nurses who are considered digital natives (Prensky, 2001) – those born between 1981 and 1996, also known as the millenial generation. However, as we noted earlier, generalisations cannot be assumed regarding generational groups. Gaughan et al. (2022) highlight a lack of skills and knowledge regarding digital technology among nurses and Reid et al. (2023) report that foundational digital skills are often not acquired during pre-registration nursing education programmes. Similarly, Kuek and Hakkennes (2020) found that although many nurses self-reported high levels of digital competence, they still experienced anxiety when using digital health technologies due to a lack of specific training. This suggests that nurses may not be adequately prepared for the level of digital skills and competence required to keep pace with rapid advances in digital health. Orhan and Kafes (2021) reported that 69.5% (139/200) of nurse participants in a cross-sectional survey believed that they were not adequately qualified to use technological devices properly and accurately.

The lack of digital literacy may have significant implications for the delivery of person-centred humanised care. Java et al. (2022) highlight that perceptions of digital health competence are intricately linked to the ability to provide care through digital channels, effectively use technology and digital health systems, and interact with patients digitally. In addition, high levels of digital literacy are associated with more positive attitudes towards the use of digital technology whereas insufficient digital literacy is associated with poor and inadequate adoption and engagement with digital health technologies (Burkoski et al., 2019). The Topol Review (Health Education England [HEE], 2019) explored how to prepare the workforce for digital transformation of healthcare and identified that, to improve digital literacy among healthcare professionals and support a digitally enabled healthcare system, digital skills training must be both integrated into healthcare education and ongoing professional development.

Future directions

This chapter has identified many of the challenges and opportunities that digitisation offers for enabling ethical, humanistic nursing care. Nurses possess critical insights into how to digital technologies can be successfully integrated and embedded within their professional ethical practice. There are three key opportunities for nurses to ensure a seamless continued digital transformation that benefits patients: (1) nurse engineers (2) digital leadership roles and (3) Patient and Public Involvement.

Nurse engineers and digital leaders

Nurse engineers play a pivotal role in the development of patient-centric digital health technologies. The full potential of these technologies is realised only when they align with patients' needs and integrate seamlessly into nurses' workflows within a framework of person-centred humanised care. It is not enough to expect nurses to simply adapt these technologies to fit into care processes while mitigating their potential dehumanising effects. No profession is better positioned than nurses to understand what is needed and effective at the point of care delivery. As such, nurse engineers are uniquely qualified to innovate and design tools that enhance nursing practice and patient care.

The role of nurse leaders in digital healthcare is evolving rapidly and is increasingly critical in harnessing digital tools to improve patient care, streamline clinical workflows, and drive innovation within healthcare systems. The ability of nurses to shape and guide digital policy and strategy for nursing practice, service delivery, healthcare teams, and organisations is only beginning to be fully recognised. What is clear, however, is that the unique skill set, and position of nurse leaders are essential and still relatively under-used in ensuring the ethical, compassionate, and patient-centred application of digital technologies.

Patient and public involvement

Meaningful patient and public involvement (PPI), as key stakeholders in designing digital healthcare solutions, is essential to ensure digital interventions both recognise and respond to the needs of communities. Within a palliative care context for example, recent PPI co-design workshops reported that when co-designing the implementation strategy for a holistic needs assessment tool active and meaningful PPI involvement, alongside other key stakeholders, led to the digital development of such a tool (Mendieta et al., 2023). Bringing all stakeholders together in this way and ensuring meaningful PPI involvement, allows researchers to co-design how they will test, evaluate and refine digital healthcare solutions that are fit for real world application. This approach can also identify key factors relating to equity as relevant to digital healthcare solutions including disparities in access and accessibility, digital literacy skills, language and cultural barriers, and financial constraints.

The implementation of healthcare interventions, such as a digital holistic needs assessment tool, is known to represent a considerable challenge within healthcare settings. Thus, active engagement of PPI as key stakeholders in designing digital healthcare solutions can allow understanding of facilitators to enable integration to promote inclusivity, equity, and minimise burden. Additionally, underpinning such activities with robust research methods contributes to evidence-based practice, the importance of which is highlighted within the literature, as contributing to improved patient outcomes and return on investment for healthcare systems (Connor et al., 2023).

Chapter summary

It is evident that digital innovation within healthcare is vast in scope and as such significantly impacts and influences nurses' professional practice. Yet in this evolution of healthcare practice, the core ethical values underpinning nursing such as equity, human and cultural rights, humanisation, and person centredness must be upheld. The digitisation of healthcare undoubtedly offers opportunities to support the delivery of person-centred care which promotes humanisation. However, if not used appropriately it can lead to dehumanised non-person-centred care. Nurses must use their advocacy role to ensure digital equity is considered within any proposed digital innovation, recognising that currently there remains a lack of universal digital access in terms of infrastructure and capability. This must be considered alongside any proposed innovation, working with people using the services (PPI) to understand any potential barriers, otherwise those with the poorest health outcomes (people who are socially excluded) will experience worsening health inequity, one of the key challenges that digital innovation seeks to address.

References

Abernethy, A., Adams, L., Barrett, M., Bechtel, C., Brennan, P., Butte, A., Faulkner, J., Fontaine, E., Friedhoff, S., Halamka, J., & Howell, M. (2022). The promise of digital health: Then, now, and the future. *NAM Perspectives*, 2022. https://doi.org/10.31478/202206e

Ali, S., Kleib, M., Paul, P., Petrovskaya, O., & Kennedy, M. (2022). Compassionate nursing care and the use of digital health technologies: A scoping review. *International Journal of Nursing Studies*, 127, 104161. https://doi.org/10.1016/j.ijnurstu.2021.104161

Alkureishi, M. A., Choo, Z. Y., Lenti, G., Castaneda, J., Zhu, M., Nunes, K., Weyer, G., Oyler, J., Shah, S., & Lee, W. W. (2021). Clinician perspectives on telemedicine: Observational cross-sectional study. *JMIR Human Factors*, 8(3), e29690. https://doi.org/10.2196/29690

Anderson, T., Prue, G., McDowell, G., Stark, P., Brown Wilson, C., Graham Wisener, L., Kerr, H., Caughers, G., Rogers, K., Cook, L., & Craig, S. (2024). Co-design and evaluation of a digital serious game to promote public awareness about pancreatic cancer. *BMC Public Health*, 24(1), 570. https://doi.org/10.1186/s12889-024-18050-7

Barnard, A., & Sandelowski, M. (2001). Technology and humane nursing care: (ir) reconcilable or invented difference? *Journal of Advanced Nursing*, 34(3), 367–375. https://doi.org/10.1046/j.1365-2648.2001.01767.x

Beauchamp, T. L., & Childress, J. F. (2001). *Principles of biomedical ethics* (5th ed.). Oxford: Oxford University Press.

Bimerew, M., & Chipps, J. (2022). Perceived technology use, attitudes, and barriers among primary care nurses. *Health SA Gesondheid*, 27, Article a2056. https://doi.org/10.4102/hsag.v27i0.2056

Boyd, D., Chang, M., & Goodman, E. (2004). Representations of digital identity. In *CSCW2004*. Available from: https://www.danah.org/papers/CSCW2004Workshop.pdf [Accessed 7.8.24].

Brown, J., Pope, N., Bosco, A. M., Mason, J., & Morgan, A. (2020). Issues affecting nurses' capability to use digital technology at work: An integrative review. *Journal of Clinical Nursing*, 29(15–16), 2801–2819. https://doi.org/10.1111/jocn.15284

Burgess, J. M., & Honey, M. (2022). Nurse leaders enabling nurses to adopt digital health: Results of an integrative literature review. *Nursing Praxis in Aotearoa New Zealand*, 38(3). https://doi.org/10.36951/001c.40333

Burkoski, V., Yoon, J., Hutchinson, D., Hall, T. N., Solomon, S., & Collins, B. E. (2019). Generational differences in hospital technology adoption: A cross-sectional study. *Nursing Leadership*, 32, 68–80. https://doi.org/10.12927/cjnl.2019.25812

Burridge, L., Foster, M., Jones, R., Geraghty, T., & Atresh, S. (2017). Person-centred care in a digital hospital: Observations and perspectives from a specialist rehabilitation setting. *Australian Health Review*, 42(5), 529–535. https://doi.org/10.1071/AH17156

Caton, E., Philippou, J., Baker, E., & Lee, G. (2024). Exploring perceptions of digital technology and digital skills among newly registered nurses and clinical managers. *Nursing Management*, 31(1). https://doi.org/10.7748/nm.2023.e2101

Connor, L., Dean, J., McNett, M., Tydings, D. M., Shrout, A., Gorsuch, P. F., Hole, A., Moore, L., Brown, R., Melnyk, B. M., & Gallagher-Ford, L. (2023). Evidence-based practice improves patient outcomes and healthcare system return on investment: Findings from a scoping review. *Worldviews on Evidence-Based Nursing*, 20(6), 6–15. https://doi.org/10.1111/wvn.12621

Department for Science Innovation and Technology. (2023). *Digital connectivity: Consultation on improving broadband for very hard to reach areas*. London: Department for Science Innovation and Technology.

Dykxhoorn, J., Osborn, D., Fischer, L., Troy, D., Kirkbride, J. B., & Walters, K. (2024). Measuring social exclusion and its distribution in England. *Social Psychiatry and Psychiatric Epidemiology*, 59(1), 187–198. https://doi.org/10.1007/s00127-023-02489-x

Ertzscheid, O. (2016). What is digital identity?: Issues, tools, methodologies (H. Tomlinson, Trans.). OpenEdition Press. Available from: https://books.openedition.org/oep/1235 [Accessed 25.7.24].

European Commission. (2024). *White paper: How to master Europe's digital infrastructure needs?* Available from: White_Paper__Ho_to_master_Europes_digital_infrastructure_needs_CkoePennGJi1hpdkuARxMGuH5s_102533 (1).pdf [Accessed 23.8.24].

Eynon, R. (2020). The myth of the digital native: Why it persists and the harm it inflicts. In T. Burns & F. Gottschalk (Eds.), *Education in the digital age: Healthy and happy children* (pp. 95–113). Paris: OECD Publishing. https://doi.org/10.1787/2dac420b-en

Farokhzadian, J., Khajouei, R., Hasman, A., & Ahmadian, L. (2020). Nurses' experiences and viewpoints about the benefits of adopting information technology in healthcare: A qualitative study in Iran. *BMC Medical Informatics and Decision Making*, 20(1), Article 240. https://doi.org/10.1186/s12911-020-01260-5

Forde-Johnston, C., Butcher, D., & Aveyard, H. (2023). An integrative review exploring the impact of electronic health records (EHR) on the quality of nurse–patient interactions and communication. *Journal of Advanced Nursing*, 79(1), 48–67. https://doi.org/10.1111/jan.15599

Friedman, J. G., Cardona Matos, Z., Szmuilowicz, E. D., & Aleppo, G. (2023). Use of continuous glucose monitors to manage type 1 diabetes mellitus: Progress, challenges, and recommendations. *Pharmacogenomics and Personalized Medicine*, 16, 263–276. https://doi.org/10.2147/PGPM.S374663

Gaughan, M. R., Kwon, M., Park, E., & Jungquist, C. (2022). Nurses' experience and perception of technology use in practice: A qualitative study using an extended technology acceptance model. *CIN: Computers, Informatics, Nursing*, 40(7), 478–486. https://doi.org/10.1097/CIN.0000000000000871

Giroux, C., & Moreau, K. (2021). A qualitative exploration of the teaching- and learning-related content nursing students share on social media. *Canadian Journal of Nursing Research*, 54(3). https://doi.org/10.1177/08445621211053113 [Accessed 23.8.24].

Gjellebæk, C., Svensson, A., Bjørkquist, C., Fladeby, N., & Grundén, K. (2020). Management challenges for future digitalization of healthcare services. *Futures*, 124, 102636. https://doi.org/10.1016/j.futures.2020.102636

Grande, D., Marti, X. L., Feuerstein-Simon, R., Merchant, R. M., Asch, D. A., Lewson, A., & Cannuscio, C. C. (2020). Health policy and privacy challenges associated with digital technology. *JAMA Network Open*, 3(7), e208285. https://doi.org/10.1001/jamanetworkopen.2020.8285

Granic, I., Morita, H., & Scholten, H. (2020). Beyond screen time: Identity development in the digital age. *Psychological Inquiry*, 31(3), 195–223. https://doi.org/10.1080/1047840X.2020.1820214

Guraya, S. S., Guraya, S. Y., & Yusoff, M. S. B. (2021). Preserving professional identities, behaviors, and values in digital professionalism using social networking sites: A systematic review. *BMC Medical Education*, 21(1), 381. https://doi.org/10.1186/s12909-021-02802-9

Health Education England (HEE). (2019). *The Topol Review: Preparing the healthcare workforce to deliver the digital future*. London: HEE.

Heaslip, V., Shannon, M., Hamilton, C., Reid, J., Oxholm, R. A., Janes, G., Phillips, N., Gentil, J., Lüdemann, B., & Langins, M. (2024). Engaging nursing and midwifery policymakers and practitioners in digital transformation: An international nursing and midwifery perspective. *BMJ Leader*. https://doi.org/10.1136/leader-2024-000990

House of Lords. (2023). *Digital exclusion: 3rd Report of session 2022–23.* House of Lords Communications and Digital Committee.

International Council of Nurses (ICN). (2021). *The ICN code of ethics for nurses.* Available from: https://www.icn.ch/sites/default/files/2023-06/ICN_Code-of-Ethics_EN_Web.pdf [Accessed 22.8.24].

Isidori, V., Diamanti, F., Gios, L., Malfatti, G., Perini, F., Nicolini, A., Longhini, J., Forti, S., Fraschini, F., Bizzarri, G., Brancorsini, S., & Gaudino, A. (2022). Digital technologies and the role of healthcare professionals: Scoping review exploring nurses' skills in the digital era and in the light of the COVID-19 pandemic. *JMIR Nursing,* 5(1), e37631. https://doi.org/10.2196/37631

Jarva, E., Oikarinen, A., Andersson, J., Tuomikoski, A. M., Kääriäinen, M., Meriläinen, M., & Mikkonen, K. (2022). Healthcare professionals' perceptions of digital health competence: A qualitative descriptive study. *Nursing Open,* 9(2), 1379–1393. https://doi.org/10.1002/nop2.1184

Janes, G., Chesterton, L., Heaslip, V., Reid, J., Lüdemann, B., Gentil, J., Oxholm, R. A., Hamilton, C., Phillips, N., & Shannon, M. (2024). Current nursing and midwifery contribution to leading digital health policy and practice: An integrative review. *Journal of Advanced Nursing.* https://doi.org/10.1111/jan.16265

Johnson, K. B., Wei, W. Q., Weeraratne, D., Frisse, M. E., Misulis, K., Rhee, K., Zhao, J., & Snowdon, J. L. (2021). Precision medicine, AI, and the future of personalized healthcare. *Clinical and Translational Science,* 14(1), 86–93. https://doi.org/10.1111/cts.12884

Kang, E. Y. N., Chen, D. R., & Chen, Y. Y. (2023). Associations between literacy and attitudes toward artificial intelligence-assisted medical consultations: The mediating role of perceived distrust and efficiency of artificial intelligence. *Computers in Human Behavior,* 139, 107529. https://doi.org/10.1016/j.chb.2022.107529

Kesavadev, J., Saboo, B., Krishna, M. B., & Krishnan, G. (2020). Evolution of insulin delivery devices: From syringes, pens, and pumps to DIY artificial pancreas. *Diabetes Therapy,* 11(6), 1251–1269. https://doi.org/10.1007/s13300-020-00831-z

Keshta, I., & Odeh, A. (2021). Security and privacy of electronic health records: Concerns and challenges. *Egyptian Informatics Journal,* 22(2), 177–183. https://doi.org/10.1016/j.eij.2020.07.003

Kings Fund. (2024). *Digital health policy timeline 1960–2016.* Available from: https://www.kingsfund.org.uk/insight-and-analysis/data-and-charts/digital-health-policy-timeline [Accessed 22.8.24].

Knop, M., Mueller, M., Kaiser, S., & Rester, C. (2024). The impact of digital technology use on nurses' professional identity and relations of power: A literature review. *Journal of Advanced Nursing,* 15(1). https://doi.org/10.1111/jan.16178

Koltsida, V., & Jonasson, L. L. (2021). Registered nurses' experiences of information technology use in home health care—From a sustainable development perspective. *BMC Nursing,* 20(1), 71. https://doi.org/10.1186/s12912-021-00602-6

Krick, T., Huter, K., Domhoff, D., Schmidt, A., Rothgang, H., & Wolf-Ostermann, K. (2019). Digital technology and nursing care: A scoping review on acceptance, effectiveness, and efficiency studies of informal and formal care technologies. *BMC Health Services Research,* 19(1), 400. https://doi.org/10.1186/s12913-019-4238-3

Kubiak, T., Priesterroth, L., & Barnard-Kelly, K. D. (2020). Psychosocial aspects of diabetes technology. *Diabetic Medicine,* 37(3), 448–454. https://doi.org/10.1111/dme.14234

Kuek, A., & Hakkennes, S. (2020). Healthcare staff digital literacy levels and their attitudes towards information systems. *Health Informatics Journal,* 26(1), 592–612. https://doi.org/10.1177/1460458219839613

Laukka, E., Hammarén, M., Pölkki, T., & Kanste, O. (2023). Hospital nurse leaders' experiences with digital technologies: A qualitative descriptive study. *Journal of Advanced Nursing*, 79(1), 297–308. https://doi.org/10.1111/jan.15466

Leonardsen, A. C. L., Bååth, C., Helgesen, A. K., Grøndahl, V. A., & Hardeland, C. (2023). Person-centeredness in digital primary healthcare services: A scoping review. *Healthcare*, 11(9), 1296. https://doi.org/10.3390/healthcare11091296

Lu, L., Zhang, J., Xie, Y., Gao, F., Xu, S., Wu, X., & Ye, Z. (2020). Wearable health devices in healthcare: Narrative systematic review. *JMIR mHealth and uHealth*, 8(11), e18907. https://doi.org/10.2196/18907

MacInnes, J., Billings, J., Coleman, A., Mikelyte, R., Croke, S., Allen, P., & Checkland, K. (2023). Scale and spread of innovation in health and social care: Insights from the evaluation of the New Care Model/Vanguard programme in England. *Journal of Health Services Research & Policy*, 28(2), 128–137. https://doi.org/10.1177/13558196221139548

MacInnes, J., Billings, J., Dima, A.L., Farmer, C., & Nijpels, G. (2021). Achieving person-centredness through technologies supporting integrated care for older people living at home: an integrative review. *Journal of Integrated Care*, 29(3), 274–294. https://doi.org/10.1108/JICA-03-2021-0013

Maslow, A. (1943). A theory of human motivation. *Psychological Review*, 50, 370–396. https://doi.org/10.1037/h0054346

McCormack, B., & McCance, T. (2021). The person-centred nursing framework. In B. McCormack & T. McCance (Eds.), *Person-centred nursing research: Methodology, methods and outcomes* (pp. 13–27). Springer International Publishing. Available from: https://content.e-bookshelf.de/media/reading/L-12873805-12a9824aea.pdf

McCormack, B., McCance, T., Bulley, C., Brown, D., McMillan, A., & Martin, S. (Eds.). (2021). *Fundamentals of person-centred healthcare practice*. John Wiley & Sons.

McCormack, B. G., Slater, P. F., Gilmour, F., Edgar, D., Gschwenter, S., McFadden, S., Hughes, C., Wilson, V., & McCance, T. (2024). The development and structural validity testing of the Person-centred Practice Inventory–Care (PCPI-C). *PLoS One*, 19(5), e0303158. https://doi.org/10.1371/journal.pone.0303158

Mendieta, C. V., de Vries, E., Calvache, J. A., Ahmedzai, S. H., Prue, G., McConnell, T., & Reid, J. (2023). Co-designing a strategy for implementing the SPARC holistic needs assessment tool in the Colombian clinical context. *Healthcare*, 11(2917). https://doi.org/10.3390/healthcare11222917

Moore, E. C., Tolley, C. L., Bates, D. W., & Slight, S. P. (2020). A systematic review of the impact of health information technology on nurses' time. *Journal of the American Medical Informatics Association*, 27(5), 798–807. https://doi.org/10.1093/jamia/ocz231

Naidu, M., & Alicia, Y. (2019). Impact of bar-code medication administration and electronic medication administration record system in clinical practice for an effective medication administration process. *Health*, 11(5), 511–526. https://doi.org/10.4236/health.2019.115044

NHS England. (2024). *NHS data model and dictionary*. Available from: https://www.datadictionary.nhs.uk/data_elements/ethnic_category.html [Accessed 23.8.24].

Office for National Statistics (ONS). (2019). *Exploring the UK's digital divide*. Available from: https://www.ons.gov.uk/peoplepopulationandcommunity/householdcharacteristics/homeinternetandsocialmediausage/articles/exploringtheuksdigitaldivide/2019-03-04 [Accessed 23.8.24].

Office for National Statistics (ONS). (2021). *What are the regional differences in income and productivity?* Available from: https://www.ons.gov.uk/visualisations/dvc1370/ [Accessed 23.8.24].

O'Kane, A., Rogers, Y., & Blandford, A. (2015). Concealing or revealing mobile medical devices? Designing for onstage and offstage presentation. In *Conference on Human*

Factors in Computing Systems (CHI-2015) (pp. 1689–1698). New York: ACM. Available from: https://www.turkiyeklinikleri.com/article/en-systematic-review-on-reengineering-digital-processes-of-healthcare-nstitutions-92979.html

Orhan, M., & Kafes, M. (2021). Systematic review on reengineering digital processes of healthcare institutions. *Turkiye Klinikleri Journal of Health Sciences*, 6(4), 973–984. Available from: https://www.turkiyeklinikleri.com/article/en-systematic-review-on-reengineering-digital-processes-of-healthcare-nstitutions-92979.html

Östman, L., Näsman, Y., Eriksson, K., & Nyström, L. (2017). Ethos: The heart of ethics and health. *Nursing Ethics*, 24(5), 568–579. https://doi.org/10.1177/0969733017695655

Owens, K., Palmore, M., Penoyer, D., & Viers, P. (2020). The effect of implementing bar-code medication administration in an emergency department on medication administration errors and nursing satisfaction. *Journal of Emergency Nursing*, 46(6), 884–891. https://doi.org/10.1016/j.jen.2020.06.011

Pickup, J. C. (2015). Technology and diabetes care: Appropriate and personalized. *Diabetic Medicine: A Journal of the British Diabetic Association*, 32(1), 3–13. https://doi.org/10.1111/dme.12559

Pinker, S. (2018). *Enlightenment now: The case for reason, science, humanism, and progress*. Viking.

Prensky, M. (2001). Digital natives, digital immigrants part 1. *On the Horizon*, 9(5), 1–6. https://doi.org/10.1108/10748120110424816

Rathert, C., Mittler, J. N., Banerjee, S., & McDaniel, J. (2017). Patient-centered communication in the era of electronic health records: What does the evidence say? *Patient Education and Counseling*, 100(1), 50–64. https://doi.org/10.1016/j.pec.2016.07.031

Reid, L., Button, D., & Brommeyer, M. (2023). Challenging the myth of the digital native: A narrative review. *Nursing Reports*, 13(2), 573–600. https://doi.org/10.3390/nursrep13020052

Sandelowski, M. (1998). Looking to care or caring to look? Technology and the rise of spectacular nursing. *Holistic Nursing Practice*, 12(4), 1–11. https://doi.org/10.1097/00004650-199807000-00004

Sharpp, T. J., Lovelace, K., Cowan, L. D., & Baker, D. (2019). Perspectives of nurse managers on information communication technology and e-leadership. *Journal of Nursing Management*, 27(7), 1554–1562. https://doi.org/10.1111/jonm.12845

Sheikh, A., Anderson, M., Albala, S., Casadei, B., Franklin, B. D., Richards, M., Taylor, D., Tibble, H., & Mossialos, E. (2021). Health information technology and digital innovation for national learning health and care systems. *The Lancet Digital Health*, 3(6), e383–e396.

Taft, T., Rudd, E. A., Thraen, I., Kazi, S., Pruitt, Z. M., Bonk, C. W., Busog, D. N., Franklin, E., Hettinger, A. Z., Ratwani, R. M., & Weir, C. R. (2023). "Are we there yet?" Ten persistent hazards and inefficiencies with the use of medication administration technology from the perspective of practicing nurses. *Journal of the American Medical Informatics Association: JAMIA*, 30(5), 809–818. https://doi.org/10.1093/jamia/ocad031

Tangari, G., Ikram, M., Ijaz, K., Kaafar, M. A., & Berkovsky, S. (2021). Mobile health and privacy: Cross-sectional study. *BMJ*, 373, n1032. https://doi.org/10.1136/bmj.n1032

Tech Partnership. (2018). *UK Consumer Digital Index 2018*. Available from: https://www.lloydsbank.com/assets/media/pdfs/banking_with_us/whats-happening/LB-Consumer-Digital-Index-2018-Report.pdf [Accessed 23.8.24].

Tin, D., Hata, R., Granholm, F., Ciottone, R. G., Staynings, R., & Ciottone, G. R. (2023). Cyberthreats: A primer for healthcare professionals. *The American Journal of Emergency Medicine*, 68, 179–185. https://doi.org/10.1016/j.ajem.2023.03.011

Todres, L., Galvin, K. T., & Holloway, I. (2009). The humanization of healthcare: A value framework for qualitative research. *International Journal of Qualitative Studies on Health and Well-Being*, 4(2), 68–77. https://doi.org/10.1080/17482620802646204

Villa-García, L., Puig, A., Puigpelat, P., Solé-Casals, M., & Fuertes, O. (2022). The development of a platform to ensure an integrated care plan for older adults with complex care needs living at home. *Journal of Integrated Care*, 30(4), 310–323. https://doi.org/10.1108/JICA-01-2022-0010

Waite, M., Aldea, A., Avari, P., Leal, Y., Martin, C., Duce, D., Fernández-Balsells, M., Fernández-Real, J. M., Herrero, P., Jugnee, N., Lui, C., López, B., Massana, J., Russell, A., Reddy, M., Wos, M., & Oliver, N. (2020). Trust and contextual engagement with the PEPPER system: The qualitative findings of a clinical feasibility study. *Journal of Diabetes Science and Technology*. Available from: https://radar.brookes.ac.uk/radar/items/784eb78c-3b05-43c8-80fa-cf0cdc603589/1

Walthall, H., Schutz, S., Snowball, J., Vagner, R., Fernandez, N., & Bartram, E. (2022). Patients' and clinicians' experiences of remote consultation: A narrative synthesis. *Journal of Advanced Nursing*, 78(7), 1954–1967. https://doi.org/10.1111/jan.15183

Wharton, G. A., Sood, H. S., Sissons, A., & Mossialos, E. (2019). Virtual primary care: Fragmentation or integration? *The Lancet Digital Health*, 1(7), e330–e331.

World Health Organization (WHO). (2016). *WHO global strategy on integrated people-centred health services 2016–2026: Placing people and communities at the centre of health services*. Available from: https://www.who.int/servicedeliverysafety/areas/people-centred-care/global-strategy/en/ [Accessed 28.8.24].

World Health Organization (WHO). (2022). *Regional digital health action plan for the WHO European Region 2023–2030*. Available from: https://www.who.int/europe/publications/i/item/EUR-RC72-5 [Accessed 22.8.24].

World Health Organization European Region. (2023). *Digital health divide: Only 1 in 2 countries in Europe and central Asia have policies to improve digital health literacy, leaving millions behind*. Available from: https://www.who.int/europe/news-room/05-09-2023-digital-health-divide--only-1-in-2-countries-in-europe-and-central-asia-have-policies-to-improve-digital-health-literacy--leaving-millions-behind [Accessed 23.8.24].

Yao, R., Zhang, W., Evans, R., Cao, G., Rui, T., & Shen, L. (2022). Inequities in health care services caused by the adoption of digital health technologies: Scoping review. *Journal of Medical Internet Research*, 24(3), e34144. https://doi.org/10.2196/34144

Yelne, S., Chaudhary, M., Dod, K., Sayyad, A., & Sharma, R. (2023). Harnessing the power of AI: A comprehensive review of its impact and challenges in nursing science and healthcare. *Cureus*, 15(11), e49252. https://doi.org/10.7759/cureus.49252

Zhang, Y., Stayt, L., Sutherland, S., & Greenway, K. (2024). How clinicians make decisions for patient management plans in telehealth. *Journal of Advanced Nursing*, 80(9), 3516–3532.

4

THE SOCIAL MEDIA NURSE

Lisa Garwood-Cross

Introduction

As the previous chapter has identified, the integration of digital technologies in healthcare has the potential to significantly reshape the landscape of nursing. However, whilst much attention has been given to the role of electronic patient record (EPR) systems, telehealth technologies and the value of apps for remote monitoring, the role of social media in nursing practice is less defined. In fact, more often than not, social media is the Aesop's fable of digital nursing practice, signalled as a warning parable of 'the nurse who posted unprofessional things on social media and got struck off'. In this context, social media becomes constructed as something for nurses to fear, a gateway to inappropriate contact from patients and potential professional ruin. Perpetuating this fear does a disservice to the potential that social media can play in professional practice and the career development of nurses. Although it is essential that nurses understand how to use social media in a considerate manner befitting their profession, this chapter argues that being aware of social media is essential for nurses in the digital age. From being able to understand the health information their patients are exposed to, through to theorising what the role of the social media nurse might be in future, this chapter encourages you to consider how social media and nursing can, and do, blur into each other's spheres of influence.

How can we define social media? While the internet was once filled with static web pages with limited interaction opportunities, over time this has evolved into a more collaborative and participatory shift, with users themselves creating content. This evolution in the way the internet is used has been referred to as 'Web 2.0', as it allowed internet users to transform from mere consumers of content and information to active contributors. This shift is the birthplace of social media. Social

DOI: 10.4324/9781032714547-4

media encompasses platforms and applications that facilitate social interaction online, usually through the creation and exchange of user-generated content. Take, for example, popular social media platforms such as Facebook, Twitter, Instagram, YouTube, and LinkedIn. If users of these platforms did not post, comment, like, share or create content, the platforms would be empty. As such, they not only enable users to connect, share various media, and interact with others' content, but rely on, and encourage, this for their survival. Social media can also include other forms of user-generated content, including forums and blogs, and direct messaging services such as WhatsApp, Messenger, KIK, and Telegram.

There has been debate over whether the transition to Web 2.0 democratises content creation and distribution by making it available to anyone with an internet connection and a device (Beer, 2009; Turner, 2006), however undoubtedly it has reshaped how information is communicated and consumed globally. As we will explore in this chapter, this continuing evolution of online information creation and exchange could have profound consequences for nurses, and thus, it is important to consider what the future might look like for the social media nurse. This chapter begins by identifying the ways in which social media may already be in the room when nurses interact with patients, exploring the influence of these digital spaces on patient-nurse interactions and trust. Following this, we will explore what it means for nurses to apply the influence their profession dictates to engage in social media spaces, and how to remain professional whilst doing so. The chapter then considers what it means to practice nursing skills in social media environments, drawing on real-life case studies of how nurses are using social media for patient benefit.

Finally, we close by theorising what the future of the social media nurse might be. How might nurses utilise social media for professional development, networking and to participate in the global exchange of nursing knowledge and expertise. Are there opportunities for nurses to practice remote care via social media to increase access to health services and what does it mean to be a nurse in an increasingly digitised social sphere?

Social media is in the room: how social media impacts nurse-patient interactions

When a patient enters a room with a clinician it is well known that it is not just the symptoms they present in the room which must be considered. Medical history, environmental factors, and many other external forces can have an impact on the health and well-being of an individual. However, for many years there was an assumption that our digital lives were somehow separate and discreet from our embodied experience in so called 'real life'. Even the common reference to non-digital interactions as 'IRL' (In Real Life) provides a reinforcement of the idea that digital interactions are somehow less 'real' or a lesser part of people's lived experience. However, our engagements and the information people consume in virtual spaces can have a very real impact on their health and well-being.

Social media platforms have been leveraged to build connections among patients with similar health conditions, creating peer-support communities (Attai et al., 2015; Dhar et al., 2018). Studies have shown that participating in these online support groups can lead to beneficial outcomes for individuals managing chronic diseases (Merolli, Gray & Martin-Sanchez, 2013). Social media health information is also easily accessible and digestible. Research by Thackery, Crookston and West (2013) indicates that approximately 75% of individuals start their healthcare information search using search engines, and about 33% have used social media sources by the time their search is complete. Social media provides patients with access to health-related information, which supports them in making well-informed decisions, increases patient empowerment (Van De Belt et al., 2010), and enables them to share their own experiences and insights, contributing user-generated content that benefits others (Kaplan & Haenlein, 2010). However, there have also been concerns raised about social media's impact on young people's mental well-being (O'Reilly et al., 2018; Ramsden & Talbot, 2024) and body image (Kleemans et al., 2018). Therefore, there is evidence that the health of patients may be directly impacted by their social media usage, both positively and negatively.

Beyond this, the COVID-19 pandemic identified that social media can also impact individuals' perception of illness and their wider trust in clinicians and healthcare systems. In times of uncertainty, such as the when the novel COVID-19 virus became known to the public, people often actively seek information to construct meaning and reduce anxiety. A study by Pengpeng, Fangqi and Qianru (2022) found that information lag from formal sources such as government and the media around COVID-19 led citizens in China to seek information from faster, informal, and unverified sources via social media. Given that social media provides opportunities for anyone to create user-generated content on fast-paced emerging topics and trends, it became a breeding ground for an excess of opinions and information related to COVID-19. This developed into what has been considered an unprecedented global 'infodemic', where an excess of information can lead to public confusion and mistrust. As Tangcharoensathien et al. (2020) note:

> The management of an infodemic becomes more challenging with social media and the rapid spread of information. Similar to epidemics, the information spreads further and faster, propagated by the interconnected ways in which information is disseminated and consumed through the web, digital and social media [...].
>
> *(p.2)*

The algorithms that underlie these platforms are trained to maximise engagement, and thus prioritise content which is often sensational, controversial or emotionally charged in nature. This environment can be particularly conducive to the spread of conspiracy theories, as individuals who show interest in such content are more likely to be recommended similar, and often more extreme, material (Bessi et al.,

2015). Because of this, algorithms can create and perpetuate echo chambers where users are repeatedly exposed to similar viewpoints, reinforcing their beliefs and increasing polarisation (Bessi et al., 2015; Bakshy et al., 2015). This is furthered as misinformation has been found to spread faster on social media than factual content (Vosoughi, Roy, & Aral, 2018). This can lead to the amplification of misleading health information (Pennycook et al., 2020; Cinelli et al., 2020) and the development of health conspiracy theories (Shahsavari et al., 2020; Allington et al., 2021) contributing to public confusion and undermining public health efforts. Concerns about social media, health misinformation, and its impact extend beyond the example of the COVID-19 pandemic. A study of 200 posts related to cancer treatment information on social media noted that 32.5% contained misinformation and 30.5% contained harmful information, furthermore this content also gained greater engagement than factual and safe content (Johnson et al., 2022). These inaccuracies can lead patients to reject evidence-based treatments in favour of ineffective and unproven alternatives, at great risk to their health (Grimes, 2022). Likewise, vaccine misinformation related to childhood immunisations, such as the disproven link between autism and vaccination, persist on social media and contribute to vaccine hesitancy among parents, leading to decreased vaccination rates and increasing susceptibility to, and prevalence of, preventable diseases (Kubin, 2019).

So why is this relevant for nurses and healthcare professionals? Given that social media has become a source of health information with the potential to impact patient health behaviours and perceptions, it cannot be assumed to be irrelevant to nursing practice. When in the room with a patient, the impact of the social media content they have consumed may also be present with them, altering their health decisions and opinion of you as a nurse. To provide patient-centred care, healthcare professionals must be aware of their patients' *information environment*, especially if they wish to enact change or counteract potential misinformation. Patients today are more informed and engaged in their healthcare decisions, often influenced by information gathered from social media. This shift requires nurses to be proficient in digital literacy to effectively guide patients in discerning reliable from unreliable health information (Moorley & Chinn, 2014). For example, Kubin (2019) highlights the importance of nurses keeping informed about the reasons families refuse or delay vaccination.

Nurses are uniquely positioned for this kind of exploratory awareness of their patients and what impacts their health literacy and decision-making, as they spend a significant amount of time with patients, building relationships and trust. Being aware of the social media landscape and content that relates to the health of your patients means that you can prepare yourself to counteract misinformation with evidence-based knowledge. In this way, if and when a patient expresses concern or distrust related to health information they have seen on social media, as a nurse you can sensitively provide discussion and evidence to help your patients navigate the confusing, overwhelming and sometimes contradictory information they have been exposed to (Sharman, 2023). Therefore, health professionals must understand the digital social media landscape to better guide and educate their patients, ensuring they receive accurate information.

Ultimately, whether we have a positive or negative view of social media, it is increasingly entering the rooms where patients and clinical staff meet, making it relevant to clinical practice. To address this, we need to expand our understanding of 'caring' to care beyond the physical nursing of wounds and illnesses, and emotional work that nurses already do so diligently, to consider the ways that nurses can become aware of these digital information ecosystems to provide an alternative, positive influence on patients, and new forms of digitally literate care.

Why do people trust social media health content? Understanding theories of health influence

When it comes to health, individuals' behaviours and decisions are rarely free from the input or influence of others. Humans are a social species and as such it is believed that our thoughts, feelings and behaviours are influenced by social connections. Traditionally, health influencers have operated within interpersonal networks, with health-related choices being shaped by influencers including family members, friends, and community leaders (Muramoto et al., 2014; Valeriani et al., 2020; Teo et al., 2019). This is often because these interpersonal relationships dictate the social norms and context of an individual, and thus their health behaviours (Amuneke-Nze, Bamgbade, & Barner, 2019). This health influence is often grounded in trust, shared experiences, and personal connections. For instance, a friend's negative experience with a specific contraceptive, e.g., a copper coil intrauterine device, might lead to a woman refusing that form of birth control, or a neighbour's encouragement to diet and exercise together might impact a person's uptake of healthy behaviours. This is why peer-education interventions have become popular as an approach to health promotion that trains peer-educators of a similar age or demographic to the target population to facilitate the teaching of health information in an attempt to utilise peer trust connections to modify health behaviours.

However, over time our spheres of influence have shifted for those who engage in social media environments. In the past, individuals might have listened to opinions or information on health by their immediate family or village. Thus, the sphere of influence on their health was small. They may have been exposed to misinformation, but the amount of misinformation exposure would be limited to the people they knew. However, for those who engage in Web 2.0 environments, where user-generated content is prevalent, a search via their phones or computers can expose them to information and opinions from hundreds of people within an hour. Often this content is created by individuals they have never met, so why might individuals trust the health information they encounter in these spaces? In some cases, exposure to repeated misinformation from multiple sources may provide the illusion of a mass of information they have uncovered, although as discussed earlier in this chapter, this may actually be because algorithms perpetuate to us the content that we previously engaged with (Jennings et al., 2021). However, some come to rely on social media health content because they have established a trust relationship with specific content creators on social media, also known as social media influencers.

To understand how these trust relationships develop we can look to the theory of Parasocial Interaction. Parasocial interaction describes a kind of psychological relationship experienced by an audience in their mediated encounters with perform-ers in the mass media and was initially developed in relation to television and film (Horton & Wohl, 1956). According to this theory, the experience of seeing a media figure repeatedly can develop a feeling as though the audience-member knows them and their life, creating an illusory experience of a social bond between them and the media figure. Of course, these interactions are typically one-sided, where the media figure neither knows the audience-member, actively participates in any interactions, nor reciprocates the relationship. Although parasocial interaction was conceived almost 70 years ago, it was in many ways before its time, in observing a phenomenon which would become central to the influencer industry more than half a century later.

Social media influencers, defined by Abidin (2016) as '*social media micro-celebrities*' have been found to instigate parasocial trust relationships from their audiences (Tolson, 2010; Cunningham & Craig, 2017). This parasocial relationship is often built through the influencers delicate balance of appearing both authentic and approachable. Authenticity has long been considered essential in the construc-tion of celebrity (Marshall, 1997), however in the influencer industry this is often constructed through specific means. For example, influencers may utilise direct to camera address, where they speak directly the audience through the camera, as though mimicking face-to-face conversation, or frequently draw attention to their ordinariness as a marker of authenticity (Tolson, 2010). Some may engage in personal disclosure and peer-led knowledge sharing (Abidin, 2019), while others position themselves as authentic everyday people situated within a community, no different from the viewers watching (Cunningham & Craig, 2017). Together, these approaches create a conversational character, which is then furthered by the ways influencers invite their audience to engage with content via commenting, direct messaging, or interactions such as Question and Answer sessions. This creates an "*unparalleled degree of interactivity between creator and fan community*" (Cun-ningham & Craig, 2017, p.74) and an aura of perceived accessibility around the influencer. It is this combination that can develop into strong parasocial bonds felt for an influencer by some of their audience members.

As influencers share their opinions and lives on social media, their perspectives on health have begun to merge into these spaces, and we have begun to see them wield their influence in relation to health (Cheng et al., 2019; Bonnevie et al., 2020; Guo et al., 2020). In addition, an increasing number of studies have identified influencers whose niche is the creation of health content, such as in the area of diet and fitness (Gil-Quintana et al., 2021; Ratwatte & Mattacola, 2021). The health content provided by social media health influencers often differs from the information patients are used to receiving from healthcare providers and other traditionally credible health sources. Whilst conventional sources favour clear and simplified clinical content, social media content offers a wide range of lived experiences, answering the more nuanced personal aspects living with illness or maintaining health. Despite many health of these influencers not being qualified health professionals (Ratwatte & Mattacola, 2021; Pilgrim & Bohnet-Joschko, 2019; Gil-Quintana et al., 2021) they instead cultivate trust from their viewers by employing the same authenticity and approachability signals discussed earlier, such as sharing their personal lives through daily vlogs where they speak directly to the camera, involving the viewer in their activities by asking questions and encouraging engagement, and developing an intimacy with the viewer by telling personal stories about their past and current lives, in relation to the health topic of fitness, and beyond (Ratwatte & Mattacola, 2021). These strategies mean that social media health influencers are also further developing the parasocial relationships their followers have with them. The average person does not see their doctor or medical teams on a weekly, or even monthly, basis. However, they might be viewing content from a social media influencer multiple times in a week or day. From this perspective, it is possible to see how and why some social media users engaging with influencer content may begin to develop trust for those sharing health information online at a faster rate than their own health professionals.

Whilst the trust social media users can develop for unqualified individuals sharing their opinions on health raises concerns about the potential for misinformation spread, this is not necessarily the death knoll for trust in healthcare professionals. It has long been considered that healthcare professionals themselves have influence over the health of their patients. Healthcare professionals can hold positions of authority and credibility in their communities due to the trust their roles and qualifications evoke. Patients rely on their expertise, turning to their doctors, nurses, and other trusted allied health professionals for advice, reassurance, and treatment recommendations. Recent studies confirm that even in the overwhelming influx of online information, a healthcare professional sharing their advice in a one-to-one setting can have significant impacts on health decision-making. A study in Singapore found that healthcare workers were important influencers in the decision-making of ambivalent older adults around influenza vaccination (Teo et al., 2019), with similar findings noted in an Australian context for encouraging parents to give the influenza vaccination for their children (Tuckerman, Crawford, & Marshall, 2020). Thus, whilst the number of voices that impact individuals' health decisions have increased dramatically since the introduction of Web 2.0, health professionals still hold a position of influence around public health.

Nursing in cyber-space: three case studies

Given that health professionals can hold a position of influence around health, what does this mean in the modern social media landscape and the opportunities it holds for nurses to expand their practice for proactive healthcare delivery? Research has suggested that to combat health-related fake news health professionals should increase their online presence (Melchior & Oliveira, 2022; Eghtesadi & Florea, 2020). Some recent studies have explored how healthcare professionals can harness social media themselves to act as online health influencers (Topf & Williams, 2021; Ngai, Singh & Lu, 2020; Zou, Zhang & Tang, 2020), including nurses (Kerr, Booth, & Jackson, 2020). By combining their professional expertise with the parasocial interaction dynamics of platforms like Instagram, TikTok, and YouTube, health professionals can reach vast audiences with health information.

Not all nurses will want to, or should be aiming to, be social media health influencers with large followings, particularly given the time commitment required and exposure this brings. However, given the need to embrace preventative care that helps to create populations engaged with managing their own health, rather than just reactive care, it is valuable to question how else nurses might be engaged in this work in digital spaces. Beyond acting as influencers, nurses can also engage in acts of nursing on social media platforms in a variety of different ways. It may be difficult for many nurses to imagine how social media environments could ever be part of the work of nursing, as our social constructions of nursing often imply that caring is a physical touch-based activity. However, caring and supporting people in digital spaces can be impactful, as we will explore in three case studies that demonstrate how nurses and midwives have been involved patient-focused communities, providing access to evidence-based health information, and informing patient-centred practice through social media.

CASE STUDY ONE: Facemums

Facemums (Chatwin et al., 2021; McCarthy et al., 2020) was a project that explored the use of midwife-moderated social media groups to provide additional antenatal support for pregnant mothers in 12 NHS trusts in the UK. *Facemums* enabled pregnant women to be referred to join private, localised, maternity-related Facebook groups. Each group had up to 20 pregnant mothers and 2 qualified midwives, who acted as moderators, within them. The midwives, referred to as '*Facewives*', provided and verified antenatal information shared within each group. This included answering specific queries the mothers identified, providing evidence-based maternity information and advice, and signposting relevant local and national services and sources of information. All *Facewives* were provided with training and mentorship to support them in delivering the service.

The project aimed to not only provide pregnant women with reliable information, but also to create virtual communities of care to support mothers, and allow them to engage in peer-support, reduce isolation and facilitate peer-to-peer information exchange. The midwives made sure that this peer exchange was done safely and without spreading misinformation by keeping an eye on the conversations among mothers in their group. When needed, they sometimes gently intervened to confirm, explain, or fix any misunderstandings or wrong or misleading information that might be shared.

In total, over 500 pregnant women and 60 midwives were involved in piloting Facemums. Research into the effectiveness of Facemum's as an intervention found it had been successful at meeting the information and support needs of pregnant women and newly delivered mothers, by improving continuity of care providing professional access to midwives and facilitating peer support in a safe and manageable way (Chatwin et al., 2021). In addition, this research noted that the *Facemums* service became a crucial resource for expectant mothers during the early stages of the COVID-19 lockdown in the UK. Data gathered to analyse the service highlighted that Facemums effectively filled the gap in antenatal support, with the *Facewives* playing a pivotal role. They verified information, managed group discussions, and provided evidence-based advice, ensuring that the service remained a trusted source of support. Their presence helped manage anxiety among members, especially when misinformation was rampant and access to regular services was limited. The *Facewives* also adapted quickly to the pressures COVID-19 put on routine local maternity services, by utilising social media functions like livestreaming to deliver trust-specific information and updates in a socially distanced manner.

The *Facemums* service was well-received, with mothers expressing that it significantly reduced their stress and anxiety. The midwives' ability to offer professional advice and verify information was particularly valued. *Facemums* not only provided a sense of community but also ensured that expectant mothers received consistent and reliable antenatal care, even during a time of uncertainty and service disruption. The service not only bridged a gap in healthcare provision but also showcased the adaptability and resilience of midwives in leveraging social media to continue delivering essential care.

The case study of *Facemums* provides us with an example of how midwives have engaged in virtual spaces to provide support to their local patients. This steps outside of the traditional boundaries of clinical and community care, by taking supportive health interventions into the digital space. What makes Facemums a particularly interesting example is the use of Facebook as a platform to engage with patients. Facebook, at the time of writing, is one of the most-used global social media platforms, by creating an intervention that utilised a digital platform that many of the expectant mothers were already using, Facemums engaged them in a space that was already comfortable for them and could bring them together to form longer-term bonds. Whilst a new platform could have been created, the use of Facebook brought health-communication and support into an app/website they were already frequenting, making it more accessible and familiar.

Midwives were integral to the success of *Facemums*, their role in the project was crucial in maintaining the quality and reliability of the service and highlights the importance of professional moderation in online health communities to provide safe and reliable information that counteracts the influx of misinformation the mothers may have been exposed to elsewhere. This case study demonstrates the potential of social media-based interventions in healthcare, with the potential for services like *Facemums* to become a staple in the future of antenatal care.

CASE STUDY TWO: The Kidney Information Network

The Kidney Information Network (KIN) is a patient-centred social media intervention designed for people living with chronic kidney disease (CKD). KIN works through a series of micro-communities run through Facebook groups that connect people with CKD to others with the same health condition in their local area (e.g., Greater Manchester, Cheshire and Merseyside, or York). The groups are designed for peer support to enable patients to network, create, and share information about living with CKD with each other and with clinicians. The Kidney Information Network also has a website which functions as a hub where patients can share blogs about their experiences, access links to both local and national kidney disease resources and find information through other social media platforms such as YouTube and Twitter.

Each KIN group is moderated by patient-moderators who maintain links with clinicians in their local trust in case they need to ask for a clinical clarification on advice. The moderators also find ways to bring together information to support the information needs of the members in their KIN groups. In addition, clinicians can join the groups to provide support and expertise, and a strong relationship between local clinical services and KIN groups has led to a range proactive health-management initiatives in the Kidney Information Network. For example, members of KIN have set up interactive Q&A events with healthcare experts from their local NHS trust to address commonly asked questions and patient concerns. These included sessions on regarding kidney-friendly dietary guidance, protective measures amid the COVID-19 outbreak, and post-transplant recover. These sessions were streamed live using video-conferencing software, as well as recorded and uploaded to the KIN Facebook page for the benefit of those who couldn't participate. Additionally, the group members established a 'healthy choices' weight management support group in collaboration with a local renal dietitian, which held virtual meetings during the COVID-19 pandemic.

Nurse Heather Jayasekera, an Advanced Renal Practitioner with over 30 years clinical experience, works as part of the Kidney Information Network team. By drawing on her extensive clinical expertise and knowledge, she supports the Kidney Information Network, picking up on cues from patients who may need additional everyday support and identifying appropriate, up-to-date information and resources that are accessible to those within the KIN communities. Her work includes identifying local and national resources, sourcing and moderating examples of 'rich, first-hand, lived experiences' of patients and their families, and interpreting guidelines that are driving renal policies and clinical practice.

When asked about how she feels about using social media as an extension of clinical practice, Heather said

> There is no doubt that social media is a key component of everyday communication. With its increasing accessibility supporting research, education and clinical practice in the health care environment it has become a powerful medium of connectivity and information that supports clinicians in a fast moving and ever-changing clinical environment. Nevertheless, it is essential that when using social media to support clinical practice, clinicians ensure that information is from a credible source and is grounded by a strong evidence base. Furthermore, users need to be aware of the legal necessity to protect themselves and their patients by recognising risks that are attached to inadvertently providing disinformation and crossing boundaries that may lead to breach of confidentiality/privacy.

Research into the impacts of the Kidney Information Network found the intervention facilitated patients access to healthcare information, aiding them to feel more informed about their condition and improve their self-management of their CKD. In addition, KIN users reported positive impacts to their well-being due to the peer-support they received from their peers and in a safe space where their frustrations, anxieties and the daily lived experience of the condition were welcomed and understood (Vasilica, et al. 2021; Vasilica, Brettle & Ormandy, 2020). Finally, the data generated from the interactions that take place in KIN groups, and questions regularly asked, are being studied by a team of researchers to understand how learnings can be made to feed back into the local renal service provision. This collaboration between the patient community and the local clinical teams fosters opportunities for the health service to continue to evolve to meet patient need.

Whilst *Facemums* is an example of a clinician-led intervention that ran for specific periods of time, the Kidney Information Network takes a more patient-led approach to long-term communities for people living with chronic kidney disease. However, part of the success of this initiative is that it involves collaboration between the patient community and local clinical teams. As the case of Heather demonstrates, there are opportunities for nurses to apply their specialist skills and knowledge to supporting patients in new and exciting ways. This support can help provide patients with the tools they need to self-manage their health better.

CASE STUDY THREE: Netnographic insights into patient experiences in nursing

Nurses can also use social media to inform patient-centred practice in different ways. Nurse Kate Covelluzzi viewed patient video blogs on YouTube to help her understand more about her patient living with the rare chronic condition Ehlers-Danlos syndrome (EDS), having never encountered the condition before. Spending the time to understand patient experiences of living with this illness provided her with a more dynamic and patient-centric understanding of the condition, informing her future interactions with people living with EDS.

Another nurse who has utilised social media to further her patient-centred practice is Stacey Munnelly, an Advanced Nurse Practitioner in Gastroenterology. Having seen firsthand the impact of chronic pancreatitis on her patients, and how painful and debilitating the condition is, Stacey wanted to raise the voices of patients in shaping understandings of supportive strategies for the illness. Noticing that patient-experience was rarely reflected in pancreatitis intervention research and following on from her work in developing pancreatitis research priorities (Munnelly et al., 2023), Stacey decided to conduct a study using social media to collect and understand the lived experience of pancreatitis patients. Using a method called netnography (Kozinets, 2020), Stacey reviewed patient blogs that chronicled their experiences of living with chronic pancreatitis, as well as engaging in Facebook groups for patients to ask questions about their experiences, and what they found helpful in relieving or managing the pain and symptoms of the condition. Using social media enabled her to reach people who might not usually take part in research and gain a detailed understanding of the stigma and tensions between patients and clinicians which cause barriers to care. Stacey is using this information gathered from social media to inform policy and practice and generate new knowledge about the experiences of pancreatitis patients to shape use of supportive strategies that will help clinicians improve care.

In comparison to the first two case studies, this example shows a different way that nurses can engage with social media as part of their nursing practice. Rather than providing information and care for patients within a virtual environment, the two nurses in this case study utilised the platforms where patients shared their lived experiences, to further their own understanding and nursing practice. This demonstrates an alternative way of centring the wisdom that can be gleamed from patient-experience.

All three of these case studies present different ways that nurses can engage in social media for the benefit of their patients and wider public health. By being present and active on social media platforms, nurses can provide evidence-based information, counteract myths, and foster a more informed public dialogue. This proactive engagement is crucial, as research indicates that content correcting mis-information can help mitigate its impact (Pennycook et al., 2020; Vosoughi, Roy, & Aral, 2018). In addition, as case study three highlights, engagement in virtual spaces can also have a positive impact on the face-to-face care nurses provide. Therefore, although there can be fear around social media use by nurses, these three case studies demonstrate the transformative potential of nurse interaction with social media initiatives for patient health.

Trust me I'm a nurse: evidence as an extension of digital professionalism

Given the casual nature of social media, and its use in personal lives, it can be easy to forget that your conduct on social media reflects on your profession. There has been much written about how nurses can stay professional online (Garwood-Cross & Haslam, 2023; Ventola, 2014). Therefore in this chapter I will not delve into the more commonly covered aspects of e-professionalism, most of which can be found by engaging with the standards and resources provided by your professional body.

Instead, it is valuable to ask, if nurses are to venture their work into the social media sphere what awareness do they need to ensure their professional practice extends suitably into these environments?

As already discussed in this chapter, professional registration as a nurse comes with an element of inbuilt public trust. However, it is known that qualification and professional registration do not guarantee that a health professional will share accurate and evidence-based information on social media. During the COVID-19 pandemic, doctors were found to have been involved in the spread of misinfor-mation, as noted by Milhazes-Cunha and Oliveira (2023) around the 'Doctors for the truth' group on Facebook that was found to spread COVID-19 misinforma-tion and conspiracy. Meanwhile, Grace (2021) notes that some nurses themselves have been involved in the spread of misinformation on social media, highlighting that although they may believe themselves fully informed, they can be subject to confirmation biases. It is unlikely that these nurses intentionally perpetuate misinformation on social media, as the nursing profession is one which is centred around protecting the health and well-being of others. Instead, more likely is that, for some, they may not have all the information on a topic or may be mistakenly misinterpreting evidence. I also do not wish to imply that anyone who thinks critically about governmental or health organisation perspectives to health should immediately be written off as perpetuating misinformation. However, a challenge in today's social media health information ecosystem is that many members of the public do not understand the nature of scientific health evidence. Given this, it is vital that any health professionals using social media for the dissemination of health information, or discussing their opinions are well versed in understanding how to engage with and communicate evidence. In embracing digital nursing in social media spaces, it is of utmost importance that nurses see being up-to-date with the evidence around the health content they share as an extension of *caring* in their nurse duties. Whilst in training pre-registration it is possible to see learning about evidence-based practice and how to interpret scientific health data as boring and unnecessary in comparison to the 'real' work of being beside. However, it is essential that nurses, and especially those who engage with health topics on social media, recognise that keeping their own knowledge updated is just as much a form of care as holding a patient's hand or inserting a nasogastric feeding tube.

Scientific evidence is paramount in guiding effective and safe health practices. When it comes to discussing health online as a nurse, while healthcare professionals often notice patterns through their anecdotal experiences, these observations should not replace peer-reviewed scientific evidence. Anecdotal experiences, although valuable in providing preliminary insights, are inherently limited by their small scale and lack of systematic methodology. Therefore, it is essential for healthcare professionals to communicate that such observations are not backed by robust evidence, underscoring the necessity for rigorously conducted research to validate any claims. By distinguishing between anecdotal observations and scientifically validated evidence, professionals can maintain credibility and ensure patient safety.

Equally important is ensuring the accurate representation of evidence-based research findings. Misrepresentation of data, whether intentional or accidental, can lead to public misinformation and unwarranted panic. For instance, reporting a 100% increase in deaths related to pineapple juice consumption without context is misleading if the actual statistic increased from one to two deaths per million people. Such misrepresentation inflates the perceived risk and can cause unnecessary alarm. Therefore, it is crucial to present health research findings in a way that accurately reflects the scale and significance of the results. This ensures that the public receives a clear and truthful understanding of health risks, enabling informed decision-making and fostering trust in the scientific community.

There are a number of tools and frameworks that can be used to aid in the evaluation of evidence and information. One of the most well-known is the CRAAP tool (Blakeslee, 2004; Lewis, 2018) which provides a simple step-by-step process for assessing sources. This can be a valuable tool to utilise before sharing health information or sources.

The future of the social media nurse

In an increasingly digital world, what might the future look like for the social media nurse? Social media offers nurses an opportunity to develop leadership skills and establish a presence in the digital healthcare community. Moorley and Chinn (2016) suggest that by leveraging platforms like Twitter and Facebook, nurse leaders can listen to individual concerns on a micro level and address them on a broader scale through data analysis and crowd sourcing. Beyond this, those who do not have formal leadership responsibilities can make use of the networking and connection opportunities afforded by social media communities of practice to amplify their voices in contributing to, and leading, discussions on important healthcare issues (Garwood-Cross & Haslam, 2023; Moorley & Chinn, 2016).This allows nurses to demonstrate their suitability for leadership via active participation in nursing communities, as well as identifying ways to continually evolve their practice through staying up to date with nursing innovation.

If social media provides a possible frontier for digital nursing, what might this look like in daily working practices of a future 'social media nurse'? As our health services take larger strides in the direction of social media, this places us at a fascinating junction to theorise the future. Let us imagine the three following fictional vignettes that demonstrate different ways that nurses might embrace the role of social media in their career:

Vignette 4.1 – Virtual MS nurse

Martin is a neurology nurse specialising in Multiple Sclerosis (MS).

He works three, 12-hour shifts per week. He spends ten hours each shift in clinical practice settings working directly with patients, and two hours per shift as a virtual MS nurse. The latter part of his role involves supporting MS patients from his local trust through a social media peer-support community and delivering online MS self-management education.

Martin enjoys the digital part of his role and finds it complements his hands-on clinical experience as he has come to understand his patients better through having an insight into their experiences. Martin shares up-to-date evidence-based research in the online community, gently correcting any misinformation he sees, and runs monthly one-hour online drop-in education sessions on managing MS.

In his role as a virtual MS nurse, Martin is exposed to a range of patient perspectives and questions. He feeds back what he finds into a quarterly update for his team on information needs so they can continue to improve their service and creates content to address those needs for both current and future patients.

Martin notices there is a new treatment for MS that is quietly being heralded as a wonder-drug, although it has not yet made national news. Martin knows that when new treatments like this are introduced to the public, his MS team are overrun with phone calls to answer questions about availability, which use a huge amount of staffing resource. So, he uses some of his virtual role time to prepare a Question & Answer (Q&A) document with a consultant in his trust about the drug, how it works, and if it will be made available to their patients. When a national newspaper runs a story about this new 'magic MS cure', Martin shares the Q&A about the drug on the peer-support community, as well as making the information available via a link on the trust website. Rather than answering the same questions repeatedly for a large number of patients, Martin's team is able to signpost to his Q&A, which results in a significant drop in calls and more time able to be spent with patients in more meaningful ways.

Vignette 4.2 – The reluctant scroller

Priyanka is an oncology nurse in Birmingham who is not a fan of social media. She doesn't like to use it in her personal life and has been guarded about its use professionally as she doesn't want to risk making any mistakes that could jeopardise her registration. However, recently Priyanka has noticed several patients making statements about how they believe they have turbo cancers caused by pesticides in industrial farming. Some of these patients are refusing evidence-based treatments as they have read on social media that switching to organic produce will remove the chemicals that are feeding their cancer, and they don't want to put any other 'poisons' in their body. Priyanka searches for journal articles about this pesticide link but cannot find any evidence to support it and is confused about the information her patients have been exposed to. She decides to join some social media platforms to understand more about her patients' perspectives and discovers a huge amount of user-generated content on TikTok and Instagram claiming to use science as the basis for their arguments. Priyanka tracks down one research paper that is named repeatedly in the posts, however on investigation she discovers that the journal later retracted the paper as it was found to have inaccuracies. Priyanka makes some notes on this topic and is able to facilitate a gentle conversation with one of her patients when he mentions the pesticide conspiracy.

Priyanka decides to use LinkedIn and X (Twitter), joining several nursing groups using hashtags such as #WeNurses to start a conversation with nursing colleagues across the country about if they have noticed any similar patterns. She is surprised to find that many colleagues in nursing and other healthcare professions respond to her posts and share parallel experiences. One nurse in Scotland reaches out to Priyanka with a resource developed by researchers on how to facilitate conversations with patients who have been exposed to online health conspiracy beliefs. Priyanka begins to use this in her own practice and finds it to be very effective at handling the matter sensitively, so she shares it with healthcare professional colleagues in her trust.

Vignette 4.3 – Social media and the school nurse

Miriam is a school nurse at Green Valley High School. Miriam has noticed that while young people often come to see her about stomach aches, they can be reluctant to ask her questions about health, particularly about contraceptives and other sensitive issues. Miriam often runs classroom sessions and assemblies but finds that getting students to engage when they are around their peers can be challenging. However, Miriam knows that many of the teenagers in her school use social media regularly. She asks a few of the more open students which platforms are popular and discovers that Instagram is highly used at GVHS. Miriam opens a dedicated Instagram page, @NurseMiriamGVSS where she shares daily health tips, reminders for vaccination schedules, and informative posts about managing common adolescent health issues, as well as posts about more taboo topics such as sex, alcohol and drugs. Miriam uses Canva to create colourful attention-grabbing health infographics and also runs an anonymous interactive Q&A session via her Instagram stories each fortnight. She ensures that her online presence is a blend of professional advice and approachable content and begins to notice that students who previously were reluctant to speak to her in person have begun to ask for advice via the direct messages on her Instagram account. Miriam always makes sure that she follows a strict code of practice in line with her professional registration but finds that allowing young people to contact her via Instagram has enabled her to meet young people's needs in an alternative way, more suited to their existing social and communication habits.

These three hypothetical examples demonstrate what embedding social media into nursing practice might look like. The examples show how social media can help nurses to support, educate, and inform patients. There are options for nurses to address health misinformation, and to connect with both other healthcare professionals and target health populations for improved patient care. The amount to which nurses wish to engage with social media will be personal to each nurse, as well as the trust they work in. However, as demonstrated in this section, there are opportunities presented by being willing to engage with social media to inform your nursing practice.

Chapter summary

Social media has become an integral part of many people's lives, influencing not only how individuals interact with each other but also how healthcare information is consumed and shared, and thus patient behaviours and expectations. Awareness of social media, and the health cultures it breeds, allows health professionals to engage with patients more effectively, as nurses must be prepared to discuss and address misconceptions that patients may bring into clinical interactions. Given the amount of time nurses spend patient-facing, compared to other healthcare professions, this awareness provides opportunities to counteract misinformation on the front line of health services.

For nurses, the intersection of social media and healthcare presents both opportunities and challenges, offering new ways to support the health of patients, but increasing the harm if incorrect information is shared. Therefore, both social media literacy and a commitment to evidence-based scholarship among nurses are crucial for the evolution of nursing practice into digital spaces. Whilst the physical aspects of nursing care will always be a central tenant of nursing practice, as this chapter has identified, there are opportunities for nurses to better the health of their patients and provide new forms of proactive healthcare delivery by engaging in social media environments.

References

Abidin, C. (2016). Visibility labour: Engaging with influencers' fashion brands and #OOTD advertorial campaigns on Instagram. *Media International Australia*, 161(1), 86–100. https://doi.org/10.1177/1329878X16665177

Abidin, C. (2019). Yes Homo: Gay influencers, homonormativity, and queerbaiting on YouTube. *Continuum*, 33(5), 614–629. https://doi.org/10.1080/10304312.2019.1644806

Allington, D., Duffy, B., Wessely, S., Dhavan, N., & Rubin, J. (2021). Health-protective behaviour, social media usage and conspiracy belief during the COVID-19 public health emergency. *Psychological Medicine*, 51(10), 1763–1769. https://doi.org/10.1017/S003329172000224X

Amuneke-Nze, C. G., Bamgbade, B. A., & Barner, J. C. (2019). An investigation of health management perceptions and wellness behaviors in African American males in central Texas. *American Journal of Men's Health*, 13(1), 1557988318813490. https://doi.org/10.1177/1557988318813490

Attai, D. J., Cowher, M. S., Al-Hamadani, M., et al. (2015). Twitter social media is an effective tool for breast cancer patient education and support: Patient-reported outcomes by survey. *Journal of Medical Internet Research*, 17(7), e188. https://doi.org/10.2196/jmir.4721

Bakshy, E., Messing, S., & Adamic, L. A. (2015). Exposure to ideologically diverse news and opinion on Facebook. *Science*, 348(6239), 1130–1132. https://doi.org/10.1126/science.aaa1160

Beer, D. (2009). Power through the algorithm? Participatory web cultures and the technological unconscious. *New Media & Society*, 11(6), 985–1002. https://doi.org/10.1177/1461444809336551

Bessi, A., Zollo, F., Del Vicario, M., Scala, A., Caldarelli, G., Stanley, H. E., & Quattrociocchi, W. (2015). Trend of narratives in the age of misinformation. *PLoS One*, 10(8), e0134641. https://doi.org/10.1371/journal.pone.0134641

Blakeslee, S. (2004). The CRAAP test. *LOEX Quarterly*, 31(3), 6–7.

Bonnevie, E., Rosenberg, S. D., Kummeth, C., Goldbarg, J., Wartella, E., & Smyser, J. (2020). Using social media influencers to increase knowledge and positive attitudes toward the flu vaccine. *PLoS One*, 15(10), e0240828. https://doi.org/10.1371/journal.pone.0240828

Chatwin, J., Butler, D., Jones, J., et al. (2021). Experiences of pregnant mothers using a social media-based antenatal support service during the COVID-19 lockdown in the UK: Findings from a user survey. *BMJ Open*, 11, e040649. https://doi.org/10.1136/bmjopen-2020-040649

Cheng, Q., Shum, A. K. Y., Ip, F. W. L., Wong, H. K., Yip, W. K. K., Kam, A. H. L., & Yip, P. S. (2019). Co-creation and impacts of a suicide prevention video. *Crisis*, 41(5), 392–399. https://doi.org/10.1027/0227-5910/a000614

Cinelli, M., Quattrociocchi, W., Galeazzi, A., Valensise, C., Brugnoli, E., Schmidt, A. L., Zola, P., Zollo, F., & Scala, A. (2020). The COVID-19 social media infodemic. *Scientific Reports*, 10(1), 16598. https://doi.org/10.1038/s41598-020-73510-5

Cunningham, S., & Craig, D. (2017). Being 'really real' on YouTube: Authenticity, community and brand culture in social media entertainment. *Media International Australia*, 164(1), 71–81. https://doi.org/10.1177/1329878X17709098

Dhar, V. K., Kim, Y., Graff, J. T., et al. (2018). Benefit of social media on patient engagement and satisfaction: Results of a 9-month, qualitative pilot study using Facebook. *Surgery*, 163(3), 565–570. https://doi.org/10.1016/j.surg.2017.09.056

Eghtesadi, M., & Florea, A. (2020). Facebook, Instagram, Reddit and TikTok: A proposal for health authorities to integrate popular social media platforms in contingency planning amid a global pandemic outbreak. *Canadian Journal of Public Health*, 111(3), 389–391. https://doi.org/10.17269/s41997-020-00343-0

https://doi.org/10.1207/S1532785XMEP0403_04

Garwood-Cross, L., & Haslam, M. (2023). Harnessing the potential of your digital collaborations. In C. Vasilica, N. Withnell, & E. Gillaspy (Eds.), *Digital skills for nursing studies and practice*. UK: SAGE.

Gil-Quintana, J., Santoveña-Casal, S., & Romero Riaño, E. (2021). Realfooders influencers on Instagram: From followers to consumers. *International Journal of Environmental Research and Public Health*, 18(4), 1624. https://doi.org/10.3390/ijerph18041624

Grace, P. J. (2021). Nurses spreading misinformation. *AJN: The American Journal of Nursing*, 121(12), 49–53. https://doi.org/10.1097/01.NAJ.0000803200.65113.fd

Grimes, D. R. (2022). The struggle against cancer misinformation. *Cancer Discovery*, 12(1), 26–30. https://doi.org/10.1158/2159-8290.CD-21-1468

Guo, M., Ganz, O., Cruse, B., Navarro, M., Wagner, D., Tate, B., & Benoza, G. (2020). Keeping it fresh with hip-hop teens: Promising targeting strategies for delivering public health messages to hard-to-reach audiences. *Health Promotion Practice*, 21(1_suppl), 61S–71S. https://journals.sagepub.com/doi/10.1177/1524839919884545

Horton, D., & Wohl, R. R. (1956). Mass communication and para-social interaction: Observations on intimacy at a distance. *Psychiatry*, 19(3), 215–229. https://doi.org/10.1080/00332747.1956.11023049

Jennings, W., Stoker, G., Bunting, H., Valgarðsson, V. O., Gaskell, J., Devine, D., & Mills, M. C. (2021). Lack of trust, conspiracy beliefs, and social media use predict COVID-19 vaccine hesitancy. *Vaccines*, 9(6), 593. https://doi.org/10.3390/vaccines9060593

Johnson, S. B., Parsons, M., Dorff, T., Moran, M. S., Ward, J. H., Cohen, S. A., & Fagerlin, A. (2022). Cancer misinformation and harmful information on Facebook and other social media: A brief report. *JNCI: Journal of the National Cancer Institute*, 114(7), 1036–1039. https://doi.org/10.1093/jnci/djac041

Kaplan, A. M., & Haenlein, M. (2010). Users of the world, unite! The challenges and opportunities of social media. *Business Horizons*, 53(1), 59–68. https://doi.org/10.1016/j.bushor.2009.09.003

Kerr, H., Booth, R., & Jackson, K. (2020). Exploring the characteristics and behaviors of nurses who have attained microcelebrity status on Instagram: Content analysis. *Journal of Medical Internet Research*, 22(5), e16540. https://doi.org/10.2196/16540

Kozinets, R. V. (2020). *Netnography: The essential guide to qualitative social media research* (3rd ed.). UK: SAGE.

Kleemans, M., Daalmans, S., Carbaat, I., & Anschütz, D. (2018). Picture perfect: The direct effect of manipulated Instagram photos on body image in adolescent girls. *Media Psychology*, 21(1), 93–110. https://doi.org/10.1080/15213269.2016.1257392

Kubin, L. (2019). Is there a resurgence of vaccine-preventable diseases in the U.S.? *Journal of Pediatric Nursing*, 44, 115–118. https://doi.org/10.1016/j.pedn.2018.11.011

Lewis, B. A. (2018). What does bad information look like? Using the CRAAP test for evaluating substandard resources. *Issues in Science and Technology Librarianship*. https://doi.org/10.5062/F41N7ZC4

Marshall, P. D. (1997). *Celebrity and power: Fame in contemporary culture*. Minneapolis: University of Minnesota Press. https://www.jstor.org/stable/10.5749/j.ctt7zw6qj

McCarthy, R., Choucri, L., Jones, J., Butler, D., Chatwin, J., Brettle, A., & Light, B. (2020). Facemums 2018: Final report. https://salford-repository.worktribe.com/preview/1503154/Facemums%20Final%20Report%20%281%29.pdf

Melchior, C., & Oliveira, M. (2022). Health-related fake news on social media platforms: A systematic literature review. *New Media & Society*, 24(6), 1500–1522. https://doi.org/10.1177/14614448211038762

Merolli, M., Gray, K., & Martin-Sanchez, F. (2013). Health outcomes and related effects of using social media in chronic disease management: A literature review and analysis of affordances. *Journal of Biomedical Informatics*, 46(6), 957–969. https://doi.org/10.1016/j.jbi.2013.04.010

Milhazes-Cunha, J., & Oliveira, L. (2023). Doctors for the truth: Echo chambers of disinformation, hate speech, and authority bias on social media. *Societies*, 13(10), 1–23.

Moorley, C., & Chinn, T. (2014). Developing nursing leadership in social media. *Journal of Advanced Nursing*, 70(3), 514–525. https://doi.org/10.1111/jan.12230

Moorley, C., & Chinn, T. (2016). Developing nursing leadership in social media. Journal of advanced nursing, 72(3), 514–520. https://doi.org/10.1111/jan.12870

Munnelly, S., Mitra, V., Leeds, J., Hopper, A., Mole, D., Philips, M., Grammatikopoulos, T., & Ryan, B., (2023). The UK top 10 research priorities from a James Lind Alliance priority setting partnership for Pancreatitis. Gastrointestinal Nursing. MA Healthcare. https://doi.org/10.12968/gasn.2024.22.1.12

Muramoto, M. L., Hall, J. R., Nichter, M., Nichter, M., Aickin, M., Connolly, T., & Lando, H. A. (2014). Activating lay health influencers to promote tobacco cessation. *American Journal of Health Behavior*, 38(3), 392–403. https://doi.org/10.5993/AJHB.38.3.10

Ngai, C. S. B., Singh, R. G., & Lu, W. (2020). Exploring drivers for public engagement in social media communication with medical social influencers in China. *PLoS One*, 15(10), e0240303. https://doi.org/10.1371/journal.pone.0240303

O'Reilly, M., Dogra, N., Whiteman, N., Hughes, J., Eruyar, S., & Reilly, P. (2018). Is social media bad for mental health and wellbeing? Exploring the perspectives of adolescents. *Clinical Child Psychology and Psychiatry*, 23(4), 601–613. https://journals.sagepub.com/doi/10.1177/1359104518775154

Pengpeng, L., Fangqi, Z., & Qianru, Z. (2022). Communication mechanisms and implications of the COVID-19 risk event in Chinese online communities. *Frontiers in Public Health*, 10, 809144. https://doi.org/10.3389/fpubh.2022.809144

Pennycook, G., McPhetres, J., Zhang, Y., Lu, J. G., & Rand, D. G. (2020). Fighting COVID-19 misinformation on social media: Experimental evidence for a scalable accuracy-nudge intervention. *Psychological Science*, 31(7), 770–780. https://doi.org/10.1177/0956797620939054

Pilgrim, K., & Bohnet-Joschko, S. (2019). Selling health and happiness: How influencers communicate on Instagram about dieting and exercise: Mixed methods research. *BMC Public Health*, 19(1), 1–9. https://doi.org/10.1186/s12889-019-7387-8

Ramsden, E., & Talbot, C. V. (2024). The role of TikTok in students' health and wellbeing. *International Journal of Mental Health and Addiction*, 1–15. https://doi.org/10.1007/s11469-023-01224-6

Ratwatte, P., & Mattacola, E. (2021). An exploration of 'fitspiration' content on YouTube and its impacts on consumers. *Journal of Health Psychology*, 26(6), 935–946. https://doi.org/10.1177/1359105319854168

Shahsavari, S., Holur, P., Wang, T., Tangherlini, T. R., & Roychowdhury, V. (2020). Conspiracy in the time of corona: Automatic detection of emerging COVID-19 conspiracy theories in social media and the news. *Journal of Computational Social Science*, 3(2), 279–317. https://doi.org/10.1007/s42001-020-00086-5

Sharman, J. (2023). Recognising and addressing health misinformation in nursing practice. *Primary Health Care*. https://doi.org/10.7748/phc.2023.e1791

Tangcharoensathien, V., Calleja, N., Nguyen, T., Purnat, T., D'Agostino, M., Garcia-Saiso, S.,..., & Briand, S. (2020). Framework for managing the COVID-19 infodemic: Methods and results of an online, crowdsourced WHO technical consultation. *Journal of Medical Internet Research*, 22(6), e19659. https://doi.org/10.2196/19659

Teo, L. M., Smith, H. E., Lwin, M. O., & Tang, W. E. (2019). Attitudes and perception of influenza vaccines among older people in Singapore: A qualitative study. *Vaccine*, 37(44), 6665–6672. https://doi.org/10.1016/j.vaccine.2019.09.049

Thackery, R., Crookston, B. T., & West, J. H. (2013). Correlates of health-related social media use among adults. *Journal of Medical Internet Research*, 15(1), e21. https://doi.org/10.2196/jmir.2297

Tolson, A. (2010). A new authenticity? Communicative practices on YouTube. *Critical Discourse Studies*, 7(4), 277–289. https://doi.org/10.1080/17405904.2010.511834

Topf, J. M., & Williams, P. N. (2021). COVID-19, social media, and the role of the public physician. *Blood Purification*, 50(4–5), 595–601. https://doi.org/10.1159/000513696

Tuckerman, J., Crawford, N. W., & Marshall, H. S. (2020). Disparities in parental awareness of children's seasonal influenza vaccination recommendations and influencers of vaccination. *PLoS One*, 15(4), e0230425. https://doi.org/10.1371/journal.pone.0230425

Turner, G. (2006). The mass production of celebrity: 'Celetoids', reality TV and the 'demotic turn'. *International Journal of Cultural Studies*, 9(2), 153–165. https://doi.org/10.1177/1367877906064028

Valeriani, G., Sarajlic Vukovic, I., Lindegaard, T., Felizia, R., Mollica, R., & Andersson, G. (2020). Addressing healthcare gaps in Sweden during the COVID-19 outbreak: On community outreach and empowering ethnic minority groups in a digitalized context. *Healthcare*, 8(4), 445. https://doi.org/10.3390/healthcare8040445

Van De Belt, T. H., Engelen, L., Berben, S. A., & Schoonhoven, L. (2010). Definition of Health 2.0 and Medicine 2.0: A systematic review. *Journal of Medical Internet Research*, 12(2), e18. https://www.jmir.org/2010/2/e18/

Vasilica, C. M., Brettle, A., & Ormandy, P. (2020). A co-designed social media intervention to satisfy information needs and improve outcomes of patients with chronic kidney disease: longitudinal study. *JMIR Formative Research*, 4(1), e13207–e13207. https://doi.org/10.2196/13207

Vasilica, C., Oates, T., Clausner, C., Ormandy, P., Barratt, J., & Graham-Brown, M. (2021). Identifying information needs of patients with iga nephropathy using an innovative social media–stepped analytical approach. *Kidney International Reports*, 6(5), 1317–1325. https://doi.org/10.1016/j.ekir.2021.02.030

Ventola, C. L. (2014). Social media and health care professionals: Benefits, risks, and best practices. *Pharmacy and Therapeutics*, 39(7), 491–499.

Vosoughi, S., Roy, D., & Aral, S. (2018). The spread of true and false news online. *Science*, 359(6380), 1146–1151. https://doi.org/10.1126/science.aap9559

Zou, W., Zhang, W. J., & Tang, L. (2020). What do social media influencers say about health? A theory-driven content analysis of top ten health influencers' posts on Sina Weibo. *Journal of Health Communication*, 26(1), 1–11. https://doi.org/10.1080/10810730.2020.1865486

5

CASE STUDY

Nursing the patient – digital technology in wound care

*Hannah Blake, Robert Douglas John Fraser
and Melanie Stephens*

Introduction

Maintaining skin integrity and treating wounds is one of the most fundamental roles of nurses. However, traditional wound care practices are now facing transformation through the use of digital technology. The purpose of this chapter is to examine digital solutions for wound prevention, assessment, monitoring, and treatment. By analysing the impact of these technologies on patient outcomes and efficiency, readers gain valuable insights into the benefits and potential limitations of incorporating digital tools into day-to-day wound care practice. Nursing theory will be applied in this context to explore how nursing care practices from educational developments can also be reimagined from a digital perspective improving outcomes for patients.

The chapter begins with introductions to the definitions of digital solutions, wound assessment, wound monitoring, and wound treatment. The chapter then examines the development of digital solutions in wound care practice. Digital solutions for wound prevention, assessment, monitoring, and treatment are explored with case studies to highlight the impact on wound care practice. Finally exploring nursing theory and education that has been reimagined from a digital perspective.

What is meant by a digital solution?

According to itransform (2024), a digital solution is a computerised method, which makes use of technology to simplify a process or solve a problem in a timelier way. These solutions can include software applications, online platforms, digital tools, and other technological innovations that aim to improve processes, enhance efficiency, and provide new opportunities for individuals and organisations. Within

DOI: 10.4324/9781032714547-5

health and care, the place, method and time care is provided is ever evolving and since the COVID-19 pandemic, in particular, there has been the development of smart health and care services, with technology being embedded across pathways, services and consultations (Crown Commercial Services, 2023). Digital transformation of health and care organisations are aiming to use technology to help health and care staff communicate better and enable people to access care more effectively and efficiently and, in a time appropriate way. Advances in medical technology are fundamental to health and care systems and can be found across the patient or service user journey from home, primary care, ambulance, hospital, and social care provision. Medical technology allows the integrated team to not only support people but understand and improve their health and care received (Department of Health and Social Care [DHSC], 2023).

Across health and care policy literature, there are definitions, categories, and classifications for medical and digital technology. The National Institute for Health and Care Excellence (2022) defines digital technologies as smartphone apps, standalone software, online tools for treating or diagnosing conditions, preventing ill health, or for improving system efficiencies and programmes that can be used to analyse data from medical devices such as scanners, sensors, or monitors. However, the framework highlights that this excludes software that is integral to, or embedded in, a medical device or in vitro diagnostic (IVD), also called software in a medical device (SiMD), technologies designed for providing training to health or care professionals (such as virtual reality [VR] or augmented reality [AR] surgical training) and technologies that facilitate data collection in research studies. The framework does, however, provide a classification and stratification of digital technologies into the tiers, based on technologies to assist in treating and diagnosing medical conditions, helping people to manage their own health and saving costs or staff time. Crucially, the framework assists innovators gather the 'correct' evidence to demonstrate their value in the UK health and social care system and to show they meet the standards set by NICE.

In comparison, the Department of Health and Social Care (2023) Medical Technology Strategy refers to digital technologies under the umbrella term of medical devices which includes those omitted in the NICE framework guidance. This includes general medical devices, active implantable medical devices (AIMDs), in vitro diagnostic medical devices (IVDs), and digital health and software. Despite these variations in definitions, categories and classifications, across the policy documents, both provide descriptions of the diverse digital technologies currently in use across health and care systems.

Definition of wound assessment, monitoring, and treatment

Wound assessment

Wound assessment is the process of obtaining vital information regarding the aetiology and physiological state of a wound through observation, questioning, physical examination, clinical investigation, and measuring of clinical features of a patient and the biopsychosocial factors to establish a baseline for planning interventions. It involves many components and is usually documented in the person's notes or care records (Nagle et al., 2023). Wound assessment tools have been developed to assist and document wound assessment processes and include tools such as the TIMERS (Tissues, Infection, Moisture, Edges, Regeneration/Repair, and Social Factors) acronym (Atkin and Tettlebach, 2019).

Wound monitoring

Wound healing is a structured process and in healthy individuals leads to restoration of the skin barrier function. However, some wounds fail to progress in a timely manner due to numerous factors either locally at the wound bed, intrinsically due to comorbidities and extrinsically from external factors such as pressure. With increasing targets such as Commissioning for Quality and Innovation (CQUINs) in the UK for pressure ulcers and lower leg wounds, there is a need to monitor interventions and treatment efficacy in wound care practices. Monitoring of the wound is therefore essential and includes knowledge of prognostic risk factors responsible for the delay in wound healing (Marques et al., 2023) and response to treatment such as change in wound size and area, wound colour changes and reduction in exudate (Dowsett, Swanson, and Karlsmark, 2019).

Wound treatment

Depending on the type of wound a person presents with, there are various treatment methods and modalities, at varying costs, available. A concept that allows health and care professionals to plan and implement care that addresses barriers to wound healing especially in hard-to-heal wounds is called wound bed preparation (WBP) (Leaper et al., 2012). It can involve many interventions from wound cleansing and debridement, prevention of infection and biofilm formation, early recognition and treatment of local infection and topical treatment options such as applying wound dressings, bandages, surgery, and instrumental methods such as negative pressure wound therapy to name but a few (Mirhaj et al., 2022).

The development of digital solutions in wound care practice

When a patient experiences a wound, there is disruption to the typical structure and function of the skin and soft tissues. To expedite the process patients will seek advice and management from nurses who practise wound care. This care is often across both the lifespan and the health and care continuum.

Across Europe an estimated 1.5–3 million people have an acute or chronic wound (Lindholm and Searle, 2016). In the UK, a point prevalence study found that 1.47 per 1,000 of the population have a complex wound (Hall et al., 2014). Globally 1%–2% of the population will experience a chronic wound within their lifetime (Falanga et al., 2022). The process of caring for people with wounds is therefore an essential part of clinical nursing practice, involving knowledge and skills of the wound healing processes, wound assessment, wound management, and referral to other services.

The skin is the largest organ, serving many critical functions. The skin protects us from the external environment and invading microorganisms. It helps with the body's thermoregulation and protects us from moisture loss. The skin helps regulate our immune system, provides sensory information, and aids the production of vitamin D. Additionally, the body has a built-in reparative process for the skin and underlying tissues that often go unnoticed when it proceeds through routine wound healing.

The wound healing process has four linear and overlapping processes: haemostasis, inflammation, proliferation, and remodelling, described in Box 1 (Falanga et al., 2022). Acute wounds move through this process in a linear fashion without significant disruption.

Wound healing phases

---

1 Haemostasis – begins immediately after injury.
2 Inflammation – begins shortly after injury and peaks three to four days post-injury; typically, complete after day 10.
3 Proliferation – begins day one post-injury and completes in 21–30 days.
4 Remodelling – begins weeks after injury and continues for up to two years.

The definition of chronic or *hard-to-heal* wounds varies. One definition includes wounds that do not progress through the normal phases of healing in a timely fashion (Falanga et al., 2022). Other definitions choose specific time markers, such as wounds that do not close in 8–12 weeks, have slow repair processes, necrotic tissues, and are possibly infected (Sili et al., 2023). Regardless of the definition, wounds that do not heal in a timely manner decrease a patients' quality of life. Chronic wounds are associated with pain and distress, negatively impact employment and social relationships, and decrease psychological well-being (Oliveira et al., 2019). Wounds also come with the risk of infection, sepsis, amputation, and mortality (Lindholm and Searle, 2016).

Across health and care settings, nurses play a critical role in wound care. This provides an opportunity to assess wound progress and escalate for more advanced treatment when the wound experiences a complication (e.g., infection), is not progressing, or the patient's needs are not being met. According to Madden and Stark (2019) advances in wound care came about when there was a shift from dry to moist wound healing. They go on to report that

a focus on the complex and multifaceted environment of chronic wound management within the aggregations of body parts, neglects social and economic determinants and contexts, relegating the impact of chronic wounds on everyday living as a secondary concern to what is happening physiologically.

(p.112)

The authors recommend that a social or public health model of patient care is required. As technology continues to transform society and the way nurses work it may offer an opportunity to enhance wound care practice and team-based care by allowing practitioners to examine the determinants of wounds within the wider context to ensure person centred care.

Historically digital technologies have been relevant to the care of patients with wounds as many organisations over time have collected audit data digitally to examine the burden of wounds to health and care resources. Chronic wounds take a long time to heal, which has required health and care professionals to examine if newer treatments and interventions are more cost effective or cost efficient, using technology to analyse and share their findings. Electronic record keeping of wound assessments, the collection of digital images of wounds and video consultation as a consequence of the COVID-19 pandemic have also meant that there has been a growth in the use of digital technologies and generation of digital data in wound care. More recently, provision of an infrastructure or reliable methods to facilitate data capture of wounds and their management has become central to the National Health Service England (NHSE) funded National Wound Care Strategy Programme (NWCSP) and US Wound Registry requiring digital technology solutions. Within wound care, the introduction of digital solutions includes many diverse applications, such as telemedicine, web-based analysis, email, mobile phones and applications, text messages, wearable devices, and clinic or remote monitoring sensors. The growth in the use of medical technology has been exponential, so much so that the annual turnover of the UK MedTech industry was reported to be £27.6 billion in 2022 (DHSC, 2023) and US $610.20bn worldwide (Statista.com., 2024).

As the use of digital technologies in wound management grows, so does the requirement that the evidence base meets service users and health and care system's needs. This includes an appraisal of the clinical effectiveness of the digital technology, the relevance to current practice, quality and robustness of the methods used to conduct the research evaluating the technology, data safety and user satisfaction of the technology, acceptability and health and digital equity, and the barriers and facilitators to implementation. A rapid scoping review by Shi et al. (2022) examined the current evidence base on the development, evaluation, and implementation of digital health technologies reported in wound care. The research team appraised the use of digital technologies for one or more of the following three functions: system level support, wound imaging and measurement, and communication. These functions were based on an adaptation of the NICE (2022, 2018) Evidence standards framework (ESF) classification system for digital technologies (see Table 5.1). One hundred and fifty-six studies were included in the review, published between 1985 and 2022. They found the most common technologies

TABLE 5.1 Functions of digital technology in wound care

Digital Health Technology Function Categories	Explanations Adapted from the NICE Evidence Standards Framework for Digital Health Technologies
System level technology	Digital health technologies that aim to improve system efficiency, including: • electronic health records (i.e., systems focusing on patients' medical history information); • decision support system (i.e., a digitalised/computerised programme for supporting judgments and care decisions in wound care); or • management systems (i.e., those focusing on operational, financial and/or clinical aspects of practice such as billing, patient registration, or triage management).
Wound imaging and measurement technologies	Digital health technologies that capture clinical data for patient monitoring. These largely include technologies for taking wound images and/or measurements. These were defined as follows. Technologies that are able to: • Capture a wound image and store it • Capture a wound image and transmit to another location • Capture a wound image and, from this, measure wound dimensions • Measure wound dimensions (without use of wound image; the technology itself does not need to capture images in the process
Communication technology	Digital health technologies that allow two-way communication between users (e.g., a video-conferencing programme for remote consultation or messaging technology).

used were wound imaging and measurement and electronic health record related function. The technologies were mainly used in acute settings and evidence was limited regarding how well the technologies are developed and implemented in practice (see Table 5.1).

Digital solutions for wound prevention

The global prevalence and healthcare costs associated with acute and chronic wounds are substantial and increasing. As healthcare shifts from a siloed secondary care model to integrated community teams across health and social care, opportunities to reduce the burden of wounds with preventative interventions using digital technology are being considered.

In a narrative review by Najafi and Mishra (2021) digital technologies supporting triaging high-risk patients, care in place, and empowering self-care in patients at risk of diabetic foot ulcers are examined. The authors report from the findings of three studies (Frykberg et al., 2017; Armstrong and Lavery, 1997; Lavery et al., 2019) that a diabetic foot prevention programme that incorporates home foot temperature and pressure monitoring may lower the incidence of ulcers in high-risk patients. They also describe the use of digital technology in the support of non-expert clinical staff in the referral of patients with diabetic foot ulcers. The use of the Society for Vascular Surgery's app "SVS iPG" (Mills et al., 2014) may assist in determining the risk of amputation and need for triage for patients with plantar foot ulcers who require timely referrals of patients.

In the prevention of pressure ulcers, an integrative review by Crotty et al. (2023) highlighted that the use of wearable sensors, worn on a patient's chest that track repositioning (turns) of the person wearing the device, are useful in the prevention of pressure ulcers as they increase staff compliance with repositioning protocols. Whilst demonstrating the usefulness of these devices, the authors also noted that the quality of the turn or repositioning of the patient was not improved. Despite this limitation, the study did present an opportunity to demonstrate the utility of wearable digital technology to assist nurses in the delivery of fundamental aspects of care.

Despite such recent advances in devices for wound prevention, during day-to-day practice, many nurses will encounter people who present with hard to heal wounds. Such wounds present a significant cost not only to health and care resources but to the person with the wound and their significant others. The next section of the chapter will explore how digital technology is assisting with wound assessment.

Digital solutions for wound assessment

To communicate important data in a timely and concise fashion, complete documentation of wound assessment is essential. However, the idea of a computerised medical record for the collation of patient data only began in the 1960s; with a clinical information system developed by Lockheed (1965) for the Mayo Clinic in Rochester. Since then, electronic medical records (EMR) have been developed to allow the capturing of a wide variety of data. Yet EMR's are only sometimes tailored to focus on wounds, creating an opportunity for various technologies to be developed to address this gap. This has included technology to track wound healing and guide clinical decision-making. In a study evaluating the use of digitisation systems in the field of chronic wound management, Reifs and colleagues (2023) identified at least ten commercially available digital wound management solutions (DWMS) with varying approvals from health regulatory bodies. Demonstrating that digital transformation of wound care is becoming more and more prevalent and part of day-to-day nursing practice.

Standardised documentation

Without standardised tools for wound assessment, wound progress towards closure is assessed through measurements, typically with a paper ruler. Length, width, and depth measurements are documentation standards. However, these methods are known to have low interrater reliability (Au et al., 2019), which complicates a clinicians' ability to determine if a wound is progressing. Furthermore, the area calculated by a length and width measurement creates a rectilinear pattern, which does not reflect the actual shape of the wound and overestimates wound size by 41% (Rogers et al., 2010). Manual measurements can perform worse on patients with darker skin tone, ill-defined wound edges, irregularly shaped wounds, and those containing nonviable tissue (Alonso et al., 2023).

Using a standardised quantitative score like the Bates-Jensen Wound Assessment Tool in a digital format, however, allows the nurse to compare scores with the previous wound assessment and identify if the current wound treatment supports healing or may require revaluation. Wound scores or wound closure can be easily tracked in graphic representation. These tools can integrate into wound care's clinical decision-making processes and escalation pathways.

The Bates-Jensen Wound Assessment Tool (BWAT) is an example of a standardised assessment tool for wound data collection (Bates-Jensen, 2022). The tool provides a numeric rating scale for 13 elements (wound size, depth, edges, undermining, necrotic tissue type, necrotic tissue amount, exudate type, exudate amount, periwound skin colour, edema, induration, granulation, and epithelisation). The score provides an output of 13–63, with higher scores representing wound degeneration and lower scores regeneration. If the wound is healed, it is scored 0.

Figure 5.1 Illustration of how a BWAT score can be integrated into wound documentation and presented to clinicians or potentially patients.

The elements of the BWAT guide structured assessment that can help direct clinical interventions to support the shift towards wound regeneration.

Wound photography

Advances in technology have changed the nature of how nurses' digital work can take place. Computers have evolved from desktop machines introduced into hospital and clinic settings, to mobile devices (e.g., smartphones and tablets) allowing nurses to bring them to the bedside and into the community. Mobile devices of today provide significant storage and computing capacity and have additional sensors such as cameras or laser-based precision measurement capability (i.e., LiDAR). In 2009, Renner et al. advocated that in addition to standardised wound assessment tools photographs should be included in the medical record to increase objective decision-making. At the time, separate digital cameras were innovative and could be uploaded from a memory card to a computer connected to the electronic medical record.

Today, smartphones create a point-of-care documentation tool that can capture images and use digital planimetry to accurately measure the surface area of the wound and track wound healing directly into the medical record (Chan and Lo, 2020). Meaning the images provide visual data that can be reviewed by a clinician, and objective data (e.g., wound size measurement) that increases documentation consistency, accuracy, and saves clinician time. These measurements can reduce the overestimation and variability of manual paper ruler measurements by

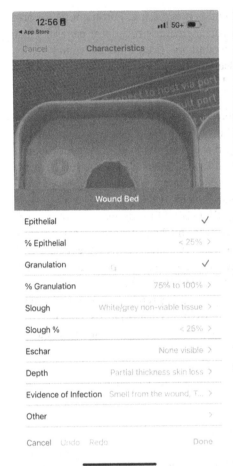
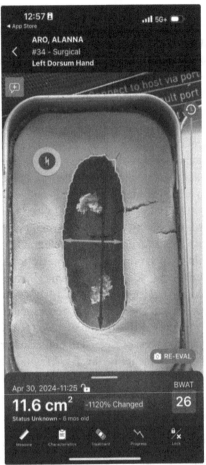

FIGURE 5.1 On the left the digital wound management solution guides clinicians through a standardised assessment tool. On the right a BWAT score can be calculated from the assessment and presented in the wound summary view for the clinician.

measuring a precise surface area, as illustrated in Figure 5.2 (Alonso et al., 2023). The green trace is the area measured through digital planimetry, and the dark and light blue lines are measures of length and width.

Digital wound measurement, when integrated into clinical processes, can also reduce time spent on measurement compared to manual methods (Mohammed et al., 2022) and collect richer data for monitoring wound progress. Surface area measurements can easily be converted to graphical trends enabling clinicians to determine the healing trajectory.

Beyond measurements, wound photography adds a rich layer of information to clinical documentation. Narrative descriptors alone make it challenging for

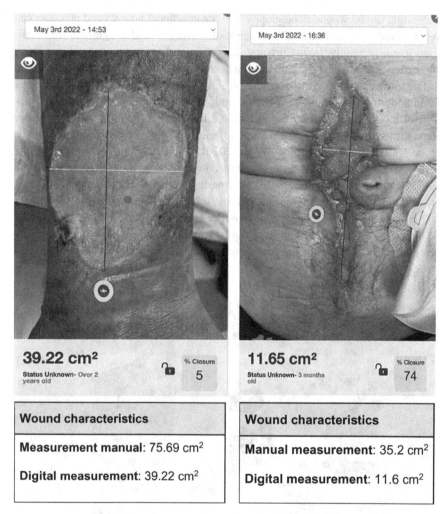

FIGURE 5.2   Comparison of digital and manual wound measurements methods.

Note: Wound photographs with patient consent courtesy of Dr. Misael Alonso. Alonso et al. (2023).

clinicians to reconstruct an accurate image and identify if the wound is progressing. For organisations considering adopting wound imaging, Onuh et al. (2022) propose an image capture algorithm:

- capture – identify the appropriate device for image capture;
- transfer – identify privacy-compliant methods for saving images to the EMR;
- storage – a secure place for storing the images, ideally in the patient record;
- analysis – images can be manually reviewed or used for artificial intelligence (AI) or data inputs; and
- utilisation – images are integrated into clinical decision-making to support patient outcomes, research, and improve documentation.

Integrating digital wound photography into organisational policies and practices can avoid privacy issues. The intuitive benefit of sharing wound images can lead clinicians to inadvertently violate privacy legislation and organisational policies using unsanctioned and unencrypted messaging or email services to transmit wound images.

Organisations must ensure policies are in place to standardise wound imaging when adopting wound photography. A study on the adoption of wound photography for monitoring the progress of diabetic foot wounds found that the two core elements that made images inadequate for clinical use were out-of-focus wounds or inadequate lighting (Anthony et al., 2020). Clinicians must be mindful of the perspective and ensure that different angles do not change the interpretation of the wound's progress (Onuh et al., 2022). Smartphone applications for wounds may provide built-in features to improve photographic wound comparison (Wang et al., 2020) or use AI to help identify wound edges or measure depth (Reifs et al., 2023).

Including digital evaluation of wounds in the medical record allows comparison over time. Reviewing images objectively reduces cognitive bias and human

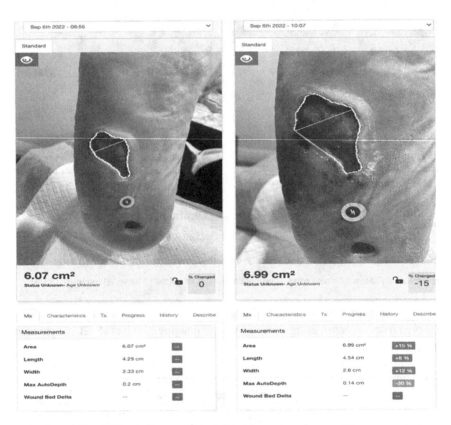

FIGURE 5.3 Comparison of pre- and post-debridement measurement.

Note: Left = predebridment, right postdebridement. Images of a wound allows comparison of measurements. Similarly, they can be used to review the healing of a wound between dressing changes. Wound photographs with patient consent courtesy of Robert Douglas John Fraser.

limitations compared to relying on clinicians' memory or narrative notes alone. This historical comparison can provide insight into the effectiveness of treatments occurring or identifying stalled wound progress (Figure 5.3). Standardised wound documentation can be compared to previous wound evaluations.

Digital solutions for wound monitoring

Vigilance in wound monitoring is essential to systematically collect, analyse, and disseminate accurate data about wound behaviour to improve healing outcomes. Poor wound monitoring can contribute to significant costs not only to health and care providers and their resources but also to the suffering of patients. As the costs and consequences of chronic wounds escalate; the ability to monitor wounds accurately through the use of digital technology can enable the collection of more sophisticated and precise information and help organisations achieve system wide improvements.

Remote digital postoperative wound monitoring

Since the COVID-19 pandemic, telehealth has become accepted and routine practice within health care (Sorensen et al., 2020). With the increase in smartphone usage, digital health interventions using this technology in surgical care are rapidly expanding. For example, a randomised controlled trial (RCT) "Tracking wound infection with smartphone technology" (TWIST) was conducted by McLean et al. (2021). The aim was to investigate whether a smartphone-delivered wound assessment tool can expedite diagnosis and treatment of surgical site infection (SSI) after emergency abdominal surgery. The authors reported that use of the smartphone demonstrated no significant difference in time-to-diagnosis of SSI. However, those using the smartphone had a higher chance of the SSI being diagnosed within seven postoperative days. The use of the smartphone also significantly reduced community care and hospital attendance with patients reporting a better experience accessing care. The researchers concluded that smartphone delivered wound follow-up is feasible, helps facilitate triage, and allows earlier postoperative diagnosis of SSI.

Wearable biosensors

Conventional wound dressings and bandages are not capable of monitoring wound healing or providing data on the behaviour and status of the wound. To address this issue researchers from California have developed wearable biosensors that provide physiological information such as the level of moisture, pressure, temperature, and pH inside a dressing or bandage (Shirzaei Sani et al., 2023). The purpose of which is to assist with monitoring wound healing. The researchers have developed a disposable wearable patch which consists of

a multimodal biosensor array for simultaneous and multiplexed electrochemical sensing of wound exudate biomarkers, a stimulus-responsive electroactive hydrogel loaded with a dual-function anti-inflammatory and antimicrobial peptide (AMP), as well as a pair of voltage-modulated electrodes for controlled drug release and electrical stimulation.

(p.2)

In vivo and in vitro evaluations have already been conducted demonstrating accelerated healing in rodents with chronic wounds. However further research is needed to demonstrate viability, safety and effectiveness in human studies.

Digital Wound Management Systems (DWMS)

To address the issue of accurate wound assessment, tissue segmentation (partitioning an image into segments corresponding to different tissue classes), and monitoring of pressure ulcers and their associated costs, skilled nursing faculty (SNF) in the US are utilising digital wound management technology (Mohammed et al., 2024). The technology is an Artificial Intelligence-powered Digital Wound Management System (DWMS) that independently identifies a wound's boundaries, measures the wound in three dimensions, and identifies tissue types using deep learning and vision architectures designed for smart devices. Data from 128 SNF's collected between 2021 and 2022 was evaluated to examine changes in PU prevalence rates, average days to healing, potential savings of clinicians' time managing PU's and applying dressings, and projected savings of out-of-pocket expenses associated with the decreased prevalence of stage 3 and 4 PU's. The findings reported that the SNF's who adopted the DWMS demonstrated reductions in days to healing, cost efficiency savings in reduced length of stay in hospital, and a reduction in the severity of PU's. Despite such positive outcomes, the researchers do acknowledge the limitations of their study including the collection of point prevalence instead of incidence data. The data collected was limited to the skilled nursing and not general settings so may not be generalisable; and there was missing data which can affect the reliability of the findings.

Case study digital solutions for wound monitoring

A Smartphone-based digital wound management app utilising AI technology to automatically calculate wound surface area, tissue type, and distribution and calculate a healing trajectory using a percentage was launched within a community healthcare setting. All staff providing wound care were issued with devices and required to complete all wound assessments via the app and attach a wound report into the EPR. This case study reflects on how the DWMS assisted with wound monitoring.

Mrs Smith was referred to a rural specialist wound care clinic, by the practice nurse, with severe arterial ulceration to her medial gaiter region, involving her Achilles tendon. A DWMS was used to monitor the progress of the wound.

The first image (Figure 5.4), taken on Mrs Smith's initial assessment, shows that the app automatically calculated the outline of the wound (following the wound edges) and the tissue distribution and classification. The clinicians identified a high

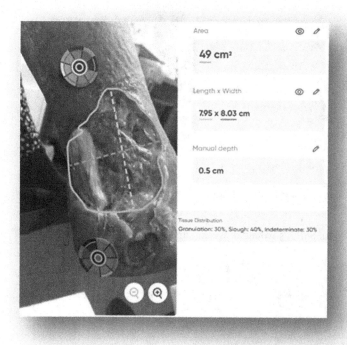

Area

49 cm²

Length x Width

7.95 x 8.03 cm

Manual depth

0.5 cm

Tissue Distribution
Granulation: 30%, Slough: 40%, Indeterminate: 30%

FIGURE 5.4   Image of Mrs Smith's wound (named changed to protect confidentiality).

bacterial burden and initiated antimicrobial treatments to help reduce infection and made onward referrals using the image captured to aid triage. From the referral, Mrs Smith received an emergency angioplasty at which point the wound healing trajectory changed and started to improve. This was shown by a reduction in wound surface area, displayed on the app for the clinicians by a wound healing percentage. The calculation of tissue distribution and classification has also changed, with a significant reduction in the percentage of slough and a sudden increase in granulation tissue, indicating that the wound has entered the proliferation phase of wound healing. The wound continued to improve over the following months and was monitored weekly by the app (Figure 5.5).

After 16 weeks, the wound was reviewed by a team member who had not seen the patient before. Mrs Smith had been experiencing increased pain around the site of the ulcer and felt that there was malodour present. Using the app, the wound assessment reported a negative wound healing trajectory, with a significant increase in wound size since the last visit (Figure 5.6). Similarly, the wound tissue classification showed 100% slough, indicative of a high bacterial burden and the wound returning to the inflammatory phase of wound healing. The team member discussed their concerns with Mrs Smith and, with consent, showed them the deterioration. Despite not knowing the patient or seeing the wound before, they were equipped with the wound data

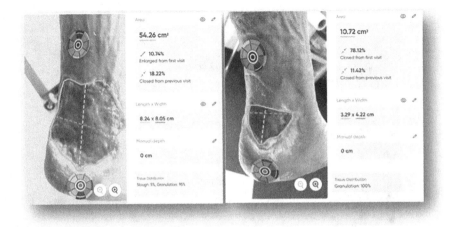

FIGURE 5.5 Mrs Smith's wound at week 4 and at week 12.

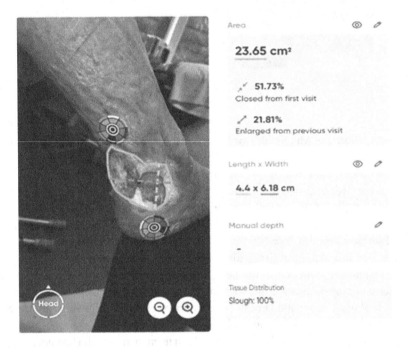

FIGURE 5.6 Mrs Smith's wound at week 16.

required at the point of care to raise a concern regarding this wound and the patient was also able to be involved in their care by sharing in this discussion. During the patient's appointment and following discussion with the patient, the team member was able to contact the senior Tissue Viability nurse who reviewed the wound remotely. Due to the data available, a decision to initiate antimicrobial dressings to help reduce the bacterial burden and associated inflammation was made.

Quote from the Tissue Viability nurse:

Before our digital wound management app, I would have no idea whether my patients' wounds were deteriorating or not improving. In order to get this information, I would have to manually search through their electronic record, calculate how long they had been receiving treatment and work out their wound size to check for deterioration or improvement, which was time-consuming. If treatments had been started, we had no standardised approach of reviewing this treatment in a timely manner, which meant that there may have been delays in optimising patient care. Similarly, if another team member wanted me to review a wound, it could take days or even weeks to get to see the patient, particularly in rural communities.

The use of the DWMS app allowed for close monitoring of Mrs Smith's wound healing trajectory and led to early identification of wound deterioration. Despite not knowing the patient, the staff member was equipped with the necessary wound data to make a decision regarding the care of this patient. The senior Tissue Viability nurse was able to provide specialist advice remotely and without delay. Whilst the patient was initially upset to see the wound deteriorating, they felt reassured that the new clinician was able to make a decision on their care immediately.

Quote from patient:

Me looking down on it looks completely different from the photo – it looked worse than it was! So, for me to see the photos all the time, it made it positive for me. I think for the staff it's great – but it's also great for the patient, because the patient can see the transformation.

Digital solutions for wound treatment

Over the last 50 years, significant advances have been made in the development of innovative dressings and efficient technologies for wound treatment. The impact of which is to hopefully accelerate healing, reduce frequency of dressing changes and improve the quality of life for those living with chronic wounds (Han and Ceilley, 2017). However, advances in digital solutions in wound treatment are still emerging.

Bioelectric bandages

For centuries bandages have been used to treat wounds such as venous leg ulcers and lymphoedema. More recently *Smart bandages* infused with electrical potential have been developed and may help with the treatment of non- healing leg wounds (Hampton and King, 2005). Reported in studies from the 1980s (Illingworth and Barker, 1980; Jaffe and Vanable, 1984) human skin has an intrinsic transepithelial potential and when there is a break in skin integrity, cells will direct the flow of ions (e.g., Na+, K+, and Cl−) through their membranes to generate an electrical current. Research suggests this plays an important role in wound healing by increasing blood flow to the wound site which, in turn, promotes fibroblast proliferation, collagen production, attraction of neutrophils, promotion, and organisation of epithelial growth (Ud-Din et al., 2012). However, a lack of studies regarding the underlying mechanism and efficacy of electrical stimulation in wound healing, has limited the development of the bandages, with most of the studies conducted in laboratories (Hosseini et al., 2021). Future clinical trials would assist in establishing the intensity, frequency, duration, and method of stimulation that may lead to their inclusion in the treatment of wounds.

Smart dressings

The properties of an ideal wound dressing have been vigorously discussed in the literature and include factors such as assisting wound closure, protection from microorganisms, the ability to absorb exudate but not dry out the wound to name but a few. Advances in material technology have enabled dressings composed of biomaterials to be responsive to ph levels, temperature, pressure, moisture, and sustained drug release. However, digital technology embedded within dressings that can have an active response to the wound status and provide tailored treatment interventions have yet to be elucidated. Laboratory studies are emerging from the literature, however more work is needed before trials in clinical settings (Rani Raju et al., 2022).

Digital solutions to assist with clinical decision-making

Transition to digital technology in day-to-day nursing practice can improve more than wound care documentation. Digital tools can allow for clinical decision support tools to be integrated and responsive to inputted data, whether this is from automated wound measurements and analysis from photographs or data entered manually by the nurse. Recent failures to embrace a systematic approach to wound management, deviations from best practice guidelines and a review highlighting new graduate nurses' wound care knowledge was insufficient (Kielo et al., 2018) have demonstrated an alternative approach to provide educational and clinical decision support at the point of care is needed. Apps utilising the World Union of Wound Healing Societies T.I.M.E. Clinical Decision Support Tool (CDST) (see Table 5.2), have been developed to support clinicians without wound care training in making better treatment decisions (for example, Smith and Nephew). The main functions of the apps allow for standardised wound assessment, a product formulary, and contextual guidance for the clinician. Evaluations of the apps have demonstrated self-reported confidence and competence with wound care practices, reductions in variations in practice and compliance with the organisations wound care formulary (Moore et al., 2022; add in others).

TABLE 5.2 Elements in T.I.M.E. clinical decision support tool

Element	Goal	Outcome
Tissue non viability	Identify necrotic tissue and slough for debridement	Viable healthy wound bed
Infection/ inflammation	Identify signs of biofilm, inflammation and infection	Noninflamed, noninfected wound
Moisture	Identify moisture level at risk of nonhealing (dry or excessive moisture)	Optimal moisture balance
Edges of wound nonadvancing	Identify non advancing wound edges	Stimulate edge advancement

Case study Digital Solutions to assist with clinical decision-making

A service evaluation by Oliver et al. (2023) examined the impact of DWMS on wound healing trajectories in patients who were found to have a deteriorating wound. Defined in the evaluation as a wound which had increased in size by over 10% from the previous digital assessment, a visual analogue pain score of >7, a new/or localised or systemic wound infection.

Across two wound care services a "senior review" process was launched, whereby a group of two or more experienced clinicians came together on a weekly basis to remotely review the wounds which had been highlighted via the DWMS as deteriorating. During these meetings care plans were optimised, which included the initiation of antimicrobial dressings, increasing compression therapy or recommending debridement techniques. The senior clinicians also made onward referrals to specialist services during these meetings to ensure that the patient was receiving optimal care.

The data from patients whose wounds were reviewed during the Senior Review meeting was then analysed to evaluate if there was an impact on wound healing rates, and compared with services which did not have a senior review process in place. Oliver and colleagues found that 56% of patients who had been reviewed via the remote Senior Review process (n = 127) had changed on to a positive wound healing trajectory, compared to 50% in all service areas without Senior Review processes (n = 894). This indicates that an extra 6% of patients benefited from the DWMS recognising their wound deterioration in combination with the remote oversight of a senior staff member optimising their treatment plan, which went on to improve their wound healing trajectory within the following weeks. It was also noted that there were wider impacts, including MDT working agreements and case-load management, which resulted in improved service delivery.

Whilst it is recognised that this evaluation has limitations, it is also recognised that improving wound healing times not only has a positive impact on patient well-being but may have cost saving and efficiency implications for service delivery.

Digital solutions to enable patient engagement in wound management practices

Integrating technology into wound care practice has been shown to improve patient engagement. Historically, the majority of patients rarely look at their wounds and rely on their clinician's opinion to monitor healing, despite how educational and motivational this act of patient empowerment may be. In a study of 71 participants who attended a wound care clinic in Toronto, Wang and colleagues (2016) examined whether the introduction of wound photography into patient monitoring fostered patient participation in wound management practices. Using a survey to elicit responses the researchers found that by encouraging patients to take photographs of their wounds on a smartphone, provided an opportunity for patients to regularly see their wound, which helped them become more involved in their care.

To further assist in patient and carer engagement DWMS have released patient versions of the application that allow wound photography, measurement and submission of questions to their care provider (Keegan et al., 2023, Kong et al., 2021). Studies evaluating the impact have demonstrated that patients can capture wound images that can be used to assess wound progress and trigger early changes in wound management (Keegan et al., 2023). Use of digital wound tracking by patients can also increase patient satisfaction due to benefits such as time and cost savings from reduced clinic-based visits (Kong et al., 2021).

Case study – Promoting engagement through continuous pressure monitoring

Pressure Ulcers are considered one of most prevalent wounds, with an estimated prevalence of around 9% of hospitalised adults (Guest et al., 2015). Pressure ulcers are considered as one of the most prevalent, avoidable harms within the NHS (NHS Improvement, 2018) and prevention alongside early recognition of patient's risk is considered key to reduce the incidence of pressure damage.

It is recognised that Pressure Ulceration can be caused by a combination of pressure, shear, and/or friction between the patient's skin and a surface (NHS Improvement, 2018). The extent of the pressure experienced through the duration of pressure in combination with the force of the pressure exerted, leads to cellular damage of the skin and deeper tissues. Generally, the level of pressure exerted at the interface (where the skin meets the surface) required to cause damage was thought to be in the region of 32 mmHg or more (Gefen, 2007), however it is similarly recognised that there is a relationship between the magnitude of pressure applied and the duration that the pressure is experienced, with larger magnitudes of pressure requiring less time to cause damage (Osuagwu et al., 2023).

A challenge faced in health and care is the recognition of when a patient is experiencing high or long levels of pressure. Tools such as the Purpose-T risk assessment tool (Coleman et al., 2018) can facilitate clinicians to assess and identify risk of PU development, but the use of a risk assessment tool cannot inform a clinician as to the level of pressure a patient is experiencing in combination with the duration. The advancement of digital technologies has allowed for new strategies to be developed with the aim of both reducing the incidence of pressure damage and improving the care and experience of patients with existing pressure damage through digital technologies, including Continuous Pressure Monitoring (CPM) (Osuagwu et al., 2023).

CPM has been used in patients with spinal injuries for many years (Fryer et al., 2023), though its role in preventing pressure ulceration across a variety of inpatient and community settings has been more recently explored (Yap et al., 2019; Caggiari et al. 2019). CPM allows clinicians to assess the patient's risk of developing pressure damage in real-time through live monitoring of the interface pressures experienced by the patient. Sensors, often in the form of a thin sheet or mat, are placed between the patient and the surface. Continuous feedback is received to a device, often a tablet, or laptop, showing the clinician the level of pressure being experienced as the surface interface. Individual squares indicate the level of pressure experienced at the surface and may be colour coded to show peaks and troughs in pressure. The sensor is often left in place for a period of 24–72 hours in order to assess the typical pressures being experienced by the patient during the day. A review by Silva et al. (2022) identified that CPM devices can also include the use of smartphone or tablet notifications to carers or clinicians, alerting them to when a patient needs to be repositioned.

CPM allows clinicians to identify areas of high or prolonged pressure, which may contribute to the risk of PU development (Fryer et al., 2023). Similarly, CPM can assist nurses to evaluate their repositioning techniques and the equipment they are using to ensure that they are facilitating the patient to be in the most comfortable and low-pressure position possible (Scott and Thurman, 2014). Without this development in digital technology, the interface pressures experienced by the patient could only have been guessed, potentially leading to unrecognised and unmanaged risk and resulting patient harm. The patient's experience of CPM has similarly indicated that the insight received through visualisation of interface pressures has helped them to engage in their treatment and better understand the need for effective repositioning (NHS Cornwall Partnership, 2021) which may to both reduce the incident of pressure damage or improve the healing of existing pressure ulcers. Silva et al. (2022) continues by highlighting the vast amount of data able to be collected through CPM may help predict a patient's risk in the future, through machine learning. They hope that retrospective patients who have gone on to develop, or avoid, pressure damage will contribute to AI technologies to help predict patient's future risk.

Digital technology and the impact on collaborative working, outcomes, and nursing efficiency

Nurses provide a significant amount of patient's wound care, yet their practice frequently involves interprofessional collaboration. Adoption of digital wound technologies facilitates communication and sharing of information with other health and care professionals, which may help improve patient experience and outcomes. Acute wounds with complications, wounds that do not heal by 30% within four weeks, and wounds that are older than 12 weeks would benefit from referral to a wound specialist (Boersema et al., 2021). Digital wound management solutions provide rich information during that referral process. An Australian initiative adopted a DWMS to support wound care quality improvement and accessibility during the COVID-19 pandemic (Barakat-Johnson et al., 2022). Nurses participating reported the ability to share images remotely to seek expert advice improved the quality of the virtual consultation and continuity of care for patients.

Leveraging digital technology can help nurses achieve better outcomes in their clinical programmes. Mohammed and colleagues (2024) noted a comprehensive wound care programme in long-term care that integrated DWMS was able to improve clinical, operational, and financial outcomes. The study looked at year over year changes in outcomes across more than 13, 291 patients. Average time to heal pressure injuries was 37% faster and the prevalence rate was 13.1% lower. Facilities received less regulator citations and penalties; an estimated 74,300 hours of nursing time was saved by better healing rates and the organisation saved $1.4 million dollars (USD) by lowering expenses related to wound care.

Digital technology and harnessing big data

A welcome benefit of the digitisation of wound care is that it can provide the opportunity for nurses to collect large amounts of clinical data on wounds. Using digital data sets nurses may have better access to information that can inform research, clinical quality improvement and the resourcing of services. Wound care nurses using digital documentation may be able to collect data on less common wounds and wound side effects. Nursing work in the future will not only be limited to practising and documenting wound care. It must incorporate research and analysis of that practice using the growing amounts of data that is digitally collected. For example, a recent study using data from a digital wound management solution published the largest prevalence study on skin tears (Fraser et al., 2022). The authors identified previous studies on skin tear prevalence used sample sizes ranging from 113 to 13,176 patients. In contrast, using the de-identified data set from the digital wound management solution a prevalence of over four years was calculated from 188,675 patients who experienced skin tears. The large sample size and data from thousands of skilled nursing facilities across North America improves the generalisability of the reported 10.3%–12.8% prevalence.

Advancing AI

Electronic documentation, standardised wound assessments, and digital photography enable nurses to adopt more advanced technologies, such as Artificial

Intelligence (AI), into clinical practice. AI can be used to perform basic tasks to improve workflow or more complex analysis aiding in care-making decisions. An AI technique called wound segmentation can automatically detect wound edges in an image, meaning clinicians do not manually identify wound edges, saving time in documentation processes (Mohammed et al., 2022). Multiple wound management solutions have demonstrated this approach and validated that it can be done using older generations of smart devices and tablets (Swerdlow et al., 2023).

Image data can be used to gather additional information. AI has been used to calculate visible depth in wounds (Anisuzzaman et al., 2022). Wounds heal from the bottom up, making insights into volume useful as these changes occur before surface closure begins in deeper wounds. Wound depth using a sterile probe can be painful for the wound and introduces potential contamination issues. It is also extremely inaccurate when calculated manually in this manner.

Tissues observed within the wound bed can provide insight into wound healing trajectories. Tissue types (e.g., eschar, granulation, slough, and epithelialisation) evolve during wounding healing. This process has a high degree of variability among clinicians depending on education, experience and skill, compared to AI, which can consistently objectively analyse tissue types in wound images (Ramachandram et al., 2022). A scoping review identified 15 studies using AI to distinguish tissue types within wound images (Dabas et al., 2023). Improved techniques to identify tissue types can help nurses focus on interpreting changes, like wound vital signs, and make appropriate follow-up decisions.

Objective wound analysis can help improve risk assessment and predictive tools. AI enables analysis of a wide variety of clinical data points within the EMR that is not feasible for clinicians to review. Gupta et al. (2024) compared AI models that identified wounds at risk of not healing and found that objective inputs performed better. These tools help clinicians focus their limited time on reviewing clients that need it most. Oota et al. (2021) used AI techniques to predict what patients required referral for speciality care for treatment and how long it would take for a wound to heal. Given the gaps identified in wound care education amongst nurses (Welsh, 2018) and human workforce challenges, AI may provide a valuable tool to nurses.

Chapter summary

Digital transformation within health and social care is challenging, as clinicians, patients and their carers engage with new ways of working. From this chapter we hope to have demonstrated that by adopting digital solutions to the prevention, assessment, monitoring, and treatment of wounds, improvements can be made in regard to communication, interprofessional working, and optimising the wound healing trajectory. Crucially, digital technologies have the capability to perform tasks which are not possible for nurses to perform effectively without these technologies. For example, wound measurement which forms the basis of the wound assessment process. These benefits, in turn, leads to positive patient outcomes, improved efficiency in service provision and patient engagement with care and recovery. The burden of wounds is set to increase with an ageing population, adopting digital technologies that optimise delivery of evidence based and clinically effective wound care could be critical. The generation of big digital datasets via the widespread use of digital technologies also offers to provide nurses with deep insights into wound healing practices and the epidemiological features of the people with wounds they care for. The case studies presented in this chapter of wounds serve as an example for what can be achieved when digital innovation is undertaken successfully in clinical nursing care.

References

Alonso, M. C., Mohammed, H. T., Fraser, R. D., Jose L. R. G. L., & Mannion, D. (2023). Comparison of wound surface area measurements obtained using clinically validated artificial intelligence-based technology versus manual methods and the effect of measurement method on debridement code reimbursement cost. *Wounds: A Compendium of Clinical Research and Practice, 35*(10), E330–E338. https://sawcs2023posters. eventscribe.net/PosterTitles.asp?PosterSortOrder=num&pfp=BrowsebyPosterNumber

Anisuzzaman, D. M., Wang, C., Rostami, B., Gopalakrishnan, S., Niezgoda, J., & Yu, Z. (2022). Image-based artificial intelligence in wound assessment: A systematic review. *Advances in Wound Care, 11*(12), 687–709.

Anthony, C. A., Femino, J. E., Miller, A. C., et al. (2020). Diabetic foot surveillance using mobile phones and automated software messaging, a randomized observational trial. *The Iowa Orthopaedic Journal, 40*(1), 35–42.

Armstrong, D. G., & Lavery, L. A. (1997). Predicting neuropathic ulceration with infrared dermal thermometry. *Journal of the American Podiatric Medical Association, 87*(7), 336–337.

Atkin, L., & Tettlebach, W. (2019). TIMERS: Expanding wound care beyond the focus of the wound. *British Journal of Nursing, 28*(20), S34–S37. https://doi.org/10.12968/bjon.2019.28.20.S34

Au, Y., Beland, B., Anderson, J. A. E., et al. (2019). Time-saving comparison of wound measurement between the ruler method and the Swift Skin and Wound App. *Journal of Cutaneous Medicine and Surgery, 23*(2), 226–228. https://doi.org/10.1177/1203475418800942

Barakat-Johnson, M., Jones, A., Burger, M., Leong, T., Frotjold, A., Randall, S., Kim, B., Fethney, J., & Coyer, F. (2022). Reshaping wound care: Evaluation of an artificial intelligence app to improve wound assessment and management amid the COVID-19 pandemic. *International Wound Journal.* https://doi.org/10.1111/iwj.13755

Bates-Jensen, B. (2022). Assessment of the patient with a wound. In L. L. McNichol, C. R. Ratliff, & S. S. Yates (Eds.), *Wound, ostomy, and continence nurses society core curriculum: Wound management* (2nd ed., pp. 55–91). Wolters Kluwer.

Boersema, G. C., Smart, H., Giaquinto-Cilliers, M. G. C., Mulder, M., Weir, G. R., Bruwer, F. A., Idensohn, P. J., Sander, J. E., Stavast, A., Swart, M., Thiart, S., & Van der Merwe, Z. (2021). Management of nonhealable and maintenance wounds: A systematic integrative review and referral pathway. *Advances in Skin & Wound Care, 34*(1), 11–22. https://doi.org/10.1097/01.ASW.0000722740.93179.9f

Caggiari, S., Worsley, P. R., & Bader, D. L. (2019). A sensitivity analysis to evaluate the performance of temporal pressure-related parameters in detecting changes in supine postures. *Medical Engineering & Physics, 69,* 33–42.

Chan, K. S., & Lo, Z. J. (2020). Wound assessment, imaging and monitoring systems in diabetic foot ulcers: A systematic review. *International Wound Journal, 17*(6), 1909–1923. https://doi.org/10.1111/iwj.13481

Coleman, S., Smith, I. L., McGinnis, E., Keen, J., Muir, D., Wilson, L., Stubbs, N., Dealey, C., Brown, S., Nelson, E. A., & Nixon, J. (2018). Clinical evaluation of a new pressure ulcer risk assessment instrument, the Pressure Ulcer Risk Primary or Secondary Evaluation Tool (PURPOSE T). *Journal of Advanced Nursing, 74*(2), 407–424.

Crotty, A., Killian, J. M., Miller, A., Chilson, S., & Wright, R. (2023). Using wearable technology to prevent pressure injuries: An integrative review. *Worldviews on Evidence-Based Nursing, 20*(4), 351–360.

Crown Commercial Services. (2023). *Digital transformation in the NHS.* https://www.crowncommercial.gov.uk/products-and-services/technology/digital-transformation-in-the-nhs

Dabas, M., Schwartz, D., Beeckman, D., Gefen, A. (2023). Application of artificial intelligence methodologies to chronic wound care and management: A scoping review. *Advances in Wound Care, 12*(4), 205–240.

Department of Health and Social Care. (2023). *Medical technology strategy.* https://assets.publishing.service.gov.uk/media/63dbe1f68fa8f57fbfff3db3/medical-technology-strategy.pdf

Dowsett, C., Swanson, T., & Karlsmark, T. (2019). A focus on the Triangle of Wound Assessment—addressing the gap challenge and identifying suspected biofilm in clinical practice. *Wounds International, 10*(3), 16–21.

Falanga, V., Isseroff, R. R., Soulika, A. M., et al. (2022). Chronic wounds. *Nature Reviews Disease Primers, 1,* 50. https://doi.org/10.1038/s41572-022-00377-3

Fraser, R. D. J., Gupta, R., & Mohammed, H. T. (2022). Analysis of real-world data from North American skilled nursing facilities' skin and wound records for skin tear prevalence, healing, and treatment. *Journal of Wound Management, 13,* 87–98.

Fryer, S., Caggiari, S., & Major, D., et al. (2023). Continuous pressure monitoring of inpatient spinal cord injured patients: Implications for pressure ulcer development. *Spinal Cord, 61,* 111–118.

Frykberg, R. G., Gordon, I. L., Reyzelman, A. M., Cazzell, S. M., Fitzgerald, R. H., Rothenberg, G. M., Bloom, J. D., Petersen, B. J., Linders, D. R., Nouvong, A., & Najafi, B. (2017). Feasibility and efficacy of a smart mat technology to predict the development of diabetic plantar ulcers. *Diabetes Care, 40*(7), 973–980.

Gefen, A. (2007). The biomechanics of sitting-acquired pressure ulcers in patients with spinal cord injury or lesions. *International Wound Journal, 4*(3), 222–231.

Guest, J. F., Ayoub, N., McIlwraith, T., Uchegbu, I., Gerrish, A., Weidlich, D., Vowden, K., & Vowden, P. (2015). Health economic burden that wounds impose on the National Health Service in the UK. *BMJ Open, 5*(12), e009283.

Gupta, R., Goldstone, L., Eisen, S., Ramachandram, D., Cassata, A., Fraser, R. D. J., Ramirez-GarciaLuna, J. L., Bartlett, R., & Allport, J. (2024). Towards an ai-based objective prognostic model for quantifying wound healing. *IEEE Journal of Biomedical And Health Informatics, 28*(2), 666–677. https://doi.org/10.1109/JBHI.2023.3251901

Hall, J., Buckley, H. L., Lamb, K. A., Stubbs, N., Saramago, P., Dumville, J. C., & Cullum, N. A. (2014). Point prevalence of complex wounds in a defined United Kingdom population. *Wound repair and regeneration: Official publication of the Wound Healing Society [and] the European Tissue Repair Society, 22*(6), 694–700. https://doi.org/10.1111/wrr.12230

Hampton, S., & King, L. (2005). Healing an intractable wound using bio-electrical stimulation therapy. *British Journal of Nursing, 14*(Sup3), S30–S32.

Han, G., & Ceilley, R. (2017). Chronic wound healing: A review of current management and treatments. *Advances in Therapy, 34*, 599–610.

Hosseini, E. S., Bhattacharjee, M., Manjakkal, L., & Dahiya, R. (2021). Healing and monitoring of chronic wounds: Advances in wearable technologies. In A. Godfrey & S. Stuart (Eds.), *Digital health* (pp. 85–99). Academic Press.

Illingworth, C. M., & Barker, A. T. (1980). Measurement of electrical currents emerging during the regeneration of amputated finger tips in children. *Clinical Physics and Physiological Measurement, 1*, 87–89.

Jaffe, L. F., & Vanable Jr, J. W. (1984). Electric fields and wound healing. *Clinics in Dermatology, 2*(3), 34–44.

Keegan, A. C., Bose, S., McDermott, K. M., Starks White, M. P., Stonko, D. P., Jeddah, D., Lev-Ari, E., Rutkowski, J., Sherman, R., Abularrage, C. J., Selvin, E., & Hicks, C. W. (2023). Implementation of a patient-centered remote wound monitoring system for management of diabetic foot ulcers. *Frontiers in Endocrinology, 14*, 1157518. https://doi.org/10.3389/fendo.2023.1157518

Kielo, E., Salminen, L., & Stolt, M. (2018). Graduating student nurses' and student podiatrists' wound care competence – An integrative literature review. *Nurse Education in Practice, 29*, 1–7. https://doi.org/10.1016/j.nepr.2017.11.002

Kong, L. Y., Ramirez-GarciaLuna, J. L., Fraser, R. D. J., & Wang, S. C. (2021). A 57-year-old man with type 1 diabetes mellitus and a chronic foot ulcer successfully managed with a remote patient-facing wound care smartphone application. *American Journal of Case Reports, 22*. https://doi.org/10.12659/AJCR.933879

Lavery, L. A., Petersen, B. J., Linders, D. R., Bloom, J. D., Rothenberg, G. M., & Armstrong, D. G. (2019). Unilateral remote temperature monitoring to predict future ulceration for the diabetic foot in remission. *BMJ Open Diabetes Research and Care, 7*(1), e000696.

Leaper, D. J., Schultz, G., Carville, K., Fletcher, J., Swanson, T., & Drake, R. (2012). Extending the TIME concept: what have we learned in the past 10 years?*. *International Wound Journal, 9*, 1–19. https://doi.org/10.1111/j.1742-481X.2012.01097.x

Lindholm, C., & Searle, R. (2016). Wound management for the 21st century: Combining effectiveness and efficiency. *International Wound Journal, 13*, 5–15. https://doi.org/10.1111/iwj.12623

Lockheed Missiles Space Company. (1965). *Hospital information system: Multihospital operational demonstration: A proposal to the United States Public Health Service*. Sunnyvale, CA: Lockheed Aircraft Corp.

Madden, M., & Stark, J. (2019). Understanding the development of advanced wound care in the UK: Interdisciplinary perspectives on care, cure, and innovation. *Journal of Tissue Viability, 28*(2), 107–114.

Marques, R., Lopes, M., Ramos, P., Neves-Amado, J., & Alves, P. (2023). Prognostic factors for delayed healing of complex wounds in adults: A scoping review. *International Wound Journal, 20*(7), 2869–2886.

McLean, K. A., Mountain, K. E., Shaw, C. A., Drake, T. M., Pius, R., Knight, S. R., Fairfield, C. J., Sgrò, A., Bouamrane, M., Cambridge, W. A., & Lyons, M. (2021). Remote diagnosis of surgical-site infection using a mobile digital intervention: A randomized controlled trial in emergency surgery patients. *NPJ Digital Medicine, 4*(1), 160.

Mills, J. L., Conte, M. S., Armstrong, D. G., Pomposelli, F. B., Schanzer, A., Sidawy, A. N., Andros, G., & Society for Vascular Surgery Lower Extremity Guidelines Committee. (2014). The Society for Vascular Surgery lower extremity threatened limb classification system: Risk stratification based on wound, ischemia, and foot infection (WIfI). *Journal of Vascular Surgery, 59*(1), 220–234.

Mirhaj, M., Labbaf, S., Tavakoli, M., & Seifalian, A. M. (2022). Emerging treatment strategies in wound care. *International Wound Journal, 19*(7), 1934–1954.

Mohammed, H. T., Bartlett, R. L., Babb, D., Fraser, R. D. J., & Mannion, D. (2022). A time motion study of manual versus artificial intelligence methods for wound assessment. *PLoS One, 17*(7), e0271742. https://doi.org/10.1371/journal.pone.0271742

Mohammed, H. T., Mannion, D., Cassata, A., & Fraser, R. D. J. (2024). Trends in pressure injury prevalence rates and average days to healing associated with adoption of a comprehensive wound care program and technology in skilled nursing facilities in the United States. *Wounds, 36*(1), 23–33.

Moore, Z. E., Aynge, G. E., Carr, C. G., Horton, A. J., Jones, H. A., Murphy, N. S., Payne, M. R., McCarthy, C. H., & Murdoch, J. M. (2022). A clinical support app for routine wound management: Reducing practice variation, improving clinician confidence and increasing formulary compliance. *International Wound Journal, 19*(5), 1263–1275.

Nagle, S. M., Stevens, K. A., & Wilbraham, S. C. (2023). Wound assessment. In *StatPearls* [Internet]. Treasure Island, FL: StatPearls Publishing. https://www.ncbi.nlm.nih.gov/books/NBK482198/

Najafi, B., & Mishra, R. (2021). Harnessing digital health technologies to remotely manage diabetic foot syndrome: A narrative review. *Medicina (Kaunas, Lithuania), 57*(4), 377. https://doi.org/10.3390/medicina57040377

National Institute for Health and Care Excellence. (2022). *Evidence standards framework for digital health technologies.* https://www.nice.org.uk/corporate/ecd7/resources/evidence-standards-framework-for-digital-health-technologies-pdf-1124017457605

NHS Cornwall Partnership. (2021). *PROMISE project.* https://www.cornwallft.nhs.uk/promise-project/

NHS Improvement. (2018). *Pressure ulcers: Revised definition and measurement.* https://www.england.nhs.uk/wp-content/uploads/2020/01/NSTPP-summary-recommendations.pdf

Oliver, M., Blake, H., Stephens, J., & Turtle-Savage, V. (2023). A formal senior review process of data from a wound management digital system to identify wounds that may be on a deteriorating trajectory: A review. *Wounds UK, 19*(4), 48–52.

Oliveira, A. C. D., Rocha, D. D. M., Bezerra, S. M. G., Andrade, E. M. L. R., Santos, A. M. R. D., & Nogueira, L. T. (2019). Quality of life of people with chronic wounds. *Acta Paulista de Enfermagem, 32*, 194–201.

Onuh, O. C., Brydges, H. T., Nasr, H., et al. (2022). Capturing essentials in wound photography past, present, and future: A proposed algorithm for standardization. *Advances in Skin & Wound Care, 35*(9), 483–492. https://doi.org/10.1097/01.ASW.0000852564.21370.a4

Oota, S. R., Rowtula, V., Mohammed, S., Galitz, J., Liu, M., & Gupta, M. (2021). Healtech-a system for predicting patient hospitalization risk and wound progression in old patients. In *Proceedings of the IEEE/CVF Winter Conference on Applications of Computer Vision* (pp. 2463–2472).

Osuagwu, B., McCaughey, E., & Purcell, M. (2023). A pressure monitoring approach for pressure ulcer prevention. *BMC Biomedical Engineering, 5*, 8.

Ramachandram, D., Ramirez-GarciaLuna, J. L., Fraser, R. D. J., Martínez-Jiménez, M. A., Arriaga-Caballero, J. E., & Allport, J. (2022). Fully automated wound tissue segmentation using deep learning on mobile devices: Cohort study. *JMIR mHealth and uHealth, 10*(4), e36977. https://doi.org/10.2196/36977

Rani Raju, N., Silina, E., Stupin, V., Manturova, N., Chidambaram, S. B., & Achar, R. R. (2022). Multifunctional and smart wound dressings—A review on recent research advancements in skin regenerative medicine. *Pharmaceutics, 14*(8), 1574.

Reifs, D., Casanova-Lozano, L., Reig-Bolaño, R., et al. (2023). Clinical validation of computer vision and artificial intelligence algorithms for wound measurement and tissue classification in wound care. *Informatics in Medicine Unlocked, 33*, 101185. https://doi.org/10.1016/j.imu.2023.101185

Rogers, L. C., Bevilacqua, N. J., Armstrong, D. G., et al. (2010). Digital planimetry results in more accurate wound measurements: A comparison to standard ruler measurements. *Journal of Diabetes Science and Technology, 4*(4), 799–802. https://doi.org/10.1177/193229681000400405

Scott, R. G., & Thurman, K. M. (2014). Visual feedback of continuous bedside pressure mapping to optimize effective patient repositioning. *Advances in Wound Care, 3*(5), 376–382.

Shi, C., Dumville, J. C., Juwale, H., Moran, C., & Atkinson, R. (2022). Evidence assessing the development, evaluation, and implementation of digital health technologies in wound care: A rapid scoping review. *Journal of Tissue Viability, 31*(4), 567–574.

Shirzaei Sani, E., Xu, C., Wang, C., Song, Y., Min, J., Tu, J., Solomon, S. A., Li, J., Banks, J. L., Armstrong, D. G., & Gao, W. (2023). A stretchable wireless wearable bioelectronic system for multiplexed monitoring and combination treatment of infected chronic wounds. *Science Advances, 9*(12), eadf7388.

Sili, A., Zaghini, F., Monaco, D., Dal Molin, A., Mosca, N., Piredda, M., & Fiorini, J. (2023). Specialized nurse-led care of chronic wounds during hospitalization and after discharge: A randomized controlled trial. *Advances in Skin & Wound Care, 36*(1), 24–29. https://doi.org/10.1097/01.ASW.0000897444.78712.fb

Silva, A., Metrôlho, J., Ribeiro, F., Fidalgo, F., & Santos, O. (2022). A review of intelligent sensor-based systems for pressure ulcer prevention. *Computers, 11*(6), 1–21.

Sorensen, M. J., Bessen, S., Danford, J., Fleischer, C., & Wong, S. L. (2020). Telemedicine for surgical consultations—Pandemic response or here to stay? A report of public perceptions. *Annals of Surgery, 272*, e174–e180.

Statista.com. (2024). *Medical technology – Worldwide.* https://www.statista.com/outlook/hmo/medical-technology/worldwide

Swerdlow, M., Lo, J., & Armstrong, D. G. (2023). Reliability of an AI-powered application across different mobile devices for assessment of chronic wounds. *Advances in Wound Care.* https://doi.org/10.1089/wound.2022.0095

Ud-Din, S., Perry, D., Giddings, P., Colthurst, J., Zaman, K., Cotton, S., Whiteside, S., Morris, J., & Bayat, A. (2012). Electrical stimulation increases blood flow and haemoglobin levels in acute cutaneous wounds without affecting wound closure time: Evidenced by non-invasive assessment of temporal biopsy wounds in human volunteers. *Experimental Dermatology, 21*(10), 758–764.

Wang, S. C., Anderson, J. A., Jones, D. V., & Evans, R. (2016). Patient perception of wound photography: Patient perception of wound photography. *International Wound Journal, 13*(3), 326–330. https://doi.org/10.1111/iwj.12293

Wang, S. C., Au, Y., & Jose, L. (2020). The promise of smartphone applications in the remote monitoring of postsurgical wounds: A literature review. *Advances in Skin & Wound Care, 33*(9), 489–496. https://doi.org/10.1097/01.ASW.0000694136.29135.02

Welsh, L. (2018). Wound care evidence, knowledge and education amongst nurses: A semi-systematic literature review. *International Wound Journal, 15*(1), 53–61. https://doi.org/10.1111/iwj.12822

Yap, T. L., Kennerly, S. M., & Ly, K. (2019). Pressure injury prevention: Outcomes and challenges to use of resident monitoring technology in a nursing home. *Journal of Wound, Ostomy, and Continence Nursing, 46*(3), 207–213.

6

CASE STUDY

Nursing the environment – digital technology in infection control

Matthew Wynn and Mark Cole

Introduction

Healthcare Associated Infection (HCAI) can be defined as an infection a patient acquires while receiving medical treatment that was not present or incubating at the time of its inception (World Health Organisation [WHO], 2011). It is the most common adverse incident experienced by people in hospital and is something that permeates all health care systems regardless of the resources available. In a modelling exercise Guest et al. (2020) estimate that in any given year there are approximately 834,000 HCAIs in the NHS and 28,500 deaths. This translates to 7.1 million occupied bed days, equivalent to 21% of the annual number of bed days across all NHS hospitals. The financial cost of HCAI is thought to exceed £2.7 billion. In addition, it is responsible for 79,700 days of absenteeism among front line Healthcare Professionals.

This chapter will focus on the intersection of digital innovation and infection prevention and control (IPC), offering a concise exploration of both the challenges and opportunities digital technologies present to IPC practices. Specifically, it will critically assess two contrasting cases: the first, an examination of digital hand hygiene monitoring systems as an example of a so far unsuccessful innovation effort, highlighting the gap between technological promise and practical application; the second, an exploration of virtual care models, showcasing a potential transformative opportunity in IPC. Through these cases, the chapter aims to underscore the importance of digital literacy among nurses, the critical role of policy and interdisciplinary collaboration in technology adoption, and the necessity of aligning digital innovations with patient-centred care principles. This focused discussion aims to navigate the complexities of integrating technology into nursing, advocating for strategic, evidence-based approaches that enhance patient outcomes while addressing the ethical, privacy, and practical challenges inherent in digital health innovations.

DOI: 10.4324/9781032714547-6

A short history of infection control

European hospitals were first established in the 12th century by religious orders and provided care for the sick, insane, and destitute. But Morbidity and Mortality was so high that typically property was disposed of, and a requiem held when the sick were admitted to a hospital (Smith et al., 2012). Despite this, sick individuals continued to congregate in hospitals that by the standards of today were crowded, dirty, poorly ventilated with multiple patients occupying a single bed. Hospital mortality was significant into the 19th century with rates of 25% common. The physician John Aiken used the phrase "hospitals are gateways to death" (Bynum, 2001). Despite this, pioneering work took place from the mid-19th century that was to transform our understanding of Microbiology, the Transmission of Disease and Infection Prevention and Control (IPC). The experiments of Louis Pasteur and Robert Koch led to what we now accept as the germ theory of disease. That is, microorganisms, too small to see with the naked eye, are responsible for certain types of disease.

At a similar point in history, Germ theory was anticipated by Ignaz Semmelweis who theorised the presence of hand-mediated cross-infection in an obstetric unit in Vienna. Semmelweis introduced a policy of handwashing, and the mortality of women dropped from 18% to 1%, Germ theory was consolidated by Joseph Lister, the father of modern surgery, who applied it to surgical techniques and wound healing with dramatic results (Michaleas et al., 2022). With Florence Nightingale, nursing witnessed its first champion in IPC. Nightingale may have lacked a scientific understanding of asepsis, and was a late adopter of the germ theory, but she recognised that a failure to apply IPC measures favoured the spread of pathogens and healthcare settings can act as amplifiers of disease during outbreaks. Her research led to the implementation of a structured programme of cleanliness and sanitation in hospitals that was to prove transformative for the profession.

Although the modern-day mantra of IPC is that it is everybody's business, nursing has invariably taken a pivotal role. In 1959, in response to a pandemic of *Staphylococcus aureus*, Dr Brendan Moore appointed an Infection Control Sister. Their role was to visit outlying hospitals and act as liaison officer for all things infection control (Perry, 2005). Due to its success, the role witnessed an exponential growth. Within ten years the newly formed infection Control Nurses Association had 71 members and within 20 years 64% of districts had appointed at least one Infection Control Nurse (ICN). By 1988, there were 205 ICNs in post in the UK. The Cooke report of 1995 then mandated that each health district should appoint at least one full-time Infection Control Nurse, and that this person should receive post-basic education. This adoption of IPC as a responsibility primarily of nurses indicates the impact of technological development, in this case the chemical technology of antibiotics, on nursing practices. It is also telling that the adoption of this responsibility was directed by the medical profession and not driven by nursing leadership. This reflects the challenges in professional role development and boundaries, which are explored in Chapter 1.

Infection control in contemporary healthcare

Despite many advances in our understanding of the transmission of disease and the IPC measures used to combat this, regrettably HCAI has not been consigned to the rear-view mirror of history. Indeed, it probably receives greater exposure and critical scrutiny than ever. In essence, the nature of HCAI has changed. Innovation has done much to improve the health of the nation, but paradoxically, this has created a society with an increasingly elderly population who have a greater prevalence of chronic disease. Advances in technology has witnessed a concomitant increase in the use of diagnostic and therapeutic procedures, broad spectrum antibiotics and immunosuppressive therapies all which compromise host defences and promote colonisation by pathogenic strains of hospital bacteria. An ageing, vulnerable population and an increase in the use of invasive procedures are then exacerbated by organisational imperatives that maximise patient flow and implement economical staff to patient ratios. The impact of these factors on the incidence of contemporary HCAI is well documented (Wilson, 2019).

Although the discipline of IPC had some appreciation of these phenomena of HCAI, it was brought into focus by a seminal study that took place in the US (Haley et al., 1985). The Study on the Efficacy of Nosocomial Infection Control (SENIC) was the most comprehensive study of HCAI undertaken to date and is widely attributed to have formed the scientific basis of IPC. SENIC was a nationwide retrospective evaluation of the cumulative index of HCAI in the US from 1970 to 1976. It spanned ten years and involved 4,000 hospitals. The study outlined the scale of HCAI and concluded that in hospitals where there was an Infection Control Programme, conducted by a nurse and one part-time physician trained in hospital epidemiology, and where specified surveillance and control guidelines were complied with, a 32% reduction of the four most common HCAI could be achieved. By contrast, in hospitals where there was no programme, and little or no compliance with specified guidelines, there was an increase in infection rates of 18% (Haley et al., 1985).

SENIC proved to be a "game changer" in the profession of IPC and activated an abundance of similar studies throughout the world, including the UK. These drew similar results and conclusions. At the heart of these findings, was that significant reductions in HCAI were possible and this would reduce morbidity and mortality, decrease lengths of stay, and reduce healthcare costs. This coincided with a highly critical National Audit Office report into the management of IPC in the NHS hospitals and public concern, fuelled by the media, of dirty hospitals and rampant flesh-eating superbugs (Brewster et al., 2016). A combination of factors meant that from 2,000 the Government made reducing the burden of HCAI a top priority. Infection Control Teams, who hitherto had operated independently were now increasingly regulated and performance managed by Central Government who produced a plethora of new legislation, guidance, and targets from 2001 to 2011.

Whether to reduce, sustain, or scale up this kind of central control is often informed by evidence of causation on key criteria. That is, do these initiatives reduce the burden of HCAI. Methicillin Resistant *Staphylococcus aureus* (MRSA) and *Clostrdioides difficle* (*C. difficile*) which are two high-profile organisms that form a part of the Department of Health's mandatory surveillance scheme. Between 2008 and 2014 MRSA bacteraemia fell by 78%, between 2007 and 2012 *C. difficile* fell by 83.9 (UK Health Security Agency, 2023). These impressive reductions have since stabilised which may suggest that incidence is now at the irreducible minimum. A point where any further reduction will be, at best, modest. Although the reductions in MRSA and *C. difficile* are welcome, attributing causation in IPC, where interventions often are multimodal and are applied in complex systems, is notoriously difficult. Nevertheless, it is plausible that the spotlight placed on HCAI at the start of the 2000, the increase in resources afforded to the IPC team, and some encouraging surveillance data, as stated above, means progress has been made, but that progress is difficult to quantify.

Looking forward

While improvements in the management of HCAI is likely, there is no sense of complacency, as HCAI, and its aetiology are intractable problems. The COVID-19 pandemic threatened the very fabric of the NHS. Moreover, a study by Knight et al. (2022) estimated that 26,600 individuals acquired a symptomatic healthcare associated SARS-CoV-2 infection in an acute Trust in England before the 31st of July 2020. This was 20.1% of all hospitalised cases. In 2016, WHO developed new guidelines to help countries combat current and future threats of infectious disease by strengthening their health service resilience at both national and facility level. The Guidelines present Core Components of Infection Prevention and Control which are a series of evidence-based and expert consensus-based recommendations that are broken down into eight core components. WHO states that these are structures that should be in place, nationally and internationally, to meet future challenges (WHO, 2016) (Table 6.1).

TABLE 6.1 WHO components of IPC

Core Component 1: IPC Programme
Core component 2: IPC guidelines
Core component 3: Education and training
Core component 4: Surveillance
Core component 5: Multimodal strategies
Core component 6: Monitoring, audit of IPC practices and feedback
Core component 6: Monitoring, audit and feedback of IPC indicators
Core component 7: Workload, staffing and bed occupancy
Core component 8: Built environment, materials and equipment at the facility level

Component one outlines how each organisation should employ an expert advisory service. Although this may be the case, a review found that there is substantial variability in IPC team structures and service delivery models (Centre for Workforce Intelligence, 2015). The IPC Professional, typically a nurse, is the clinical facing part of the team and is expected to work at an advanced practice level. However, there is no clearly defined pathway into IPC and the role has no baseline qualification. There is no uniformity in person specifications and the role has different remits and responsibilities depending on the organisation.

The second component recognises the importance of evidence-based guidelines. There are a vast number of IPC guidelines that have been produced by national and international government and professional organisations. These clinical guidelines serve several purposes including improving the effectiveness and quality of care, reducing variations in healthcare practices as well as decreasing costly and avoidable adverse events (Mitchell, 2020). But providing high-quality guidelines does not necessarily lead to a change in clinical practice. A review by Pereira et al. (2022) concluded that the successful introduction of guidelines involves three steps, development, dissemination, and implementation. Often it is not the development phase that is the point of breakdown, but how they are disseminated. That is how they are brought to the consciousness of a time poor, busy healthcare worker.

IPC education for all healthcare workers is the third component of the framework. A systematic review into knowledge of IPC and compliance proposed knowledge is essential for effective IPC. Deficient understanding of IPC guidelines, risks of infection and modes of transmission, coupled with a lack of understanding on the appropriateness, efficacy, and use of IPC measure can all become barriers to compliance (Alhumaid et al., 2021). Nonetheless, it would be wrong to assume that there is a direct, linear relationship between education, knowledge, and practice. There are many other confounding variables that may determine behaviour. Education and knowledge may be the cornerstone of practice, but they are best seen as a foundation, something to be built upon, rather than end in and of itself. WHO advocate that education should innovative, multifactorial, participatory, and should include simulation (WHO, 2016).

Component 4 has its focus on surveillance, defined as the "ongoing systematic collection and analysis, interpretation, and dissemination of data regarding a healthcare event for use to reduce morbidity, mortality, and to improve health" (Centres for Disease Control and Prevention, 2001). In the UK, the surveillance activities of IPC teams tend to be directed at the capture of data to meet national imperatives. Involvement in the analysis, dissemination, and application is limited as this tends to occur at a national rather than a local level. Ridelberg and Nilsen (2015) interviewed a group of IPC professionals about their abilities to conduct their own surveillance. The cohort raised several concerns, including their technical skills, epidemiological competence, quality of the software, relevance of the data, competence, and their time to conduct their own local, meaningful, surveillance data. In relation to workload, they noted that opportunities may exist to improve efficiency through greater use of technologies to interrogate data that is already routinely available in hospital electronic databases.

Component 5 introduces the notion of multi modals strategies. A multimodal strategy is best described as several elements (three or more; usually five) that are implemented in an integrated way to guide action and provide focus (Lavellee et al., 2017). It is based on the premise that behaviour change is complex and if you only target a single area this is likely to result in failure. The classic WHO multi modal approach to IPC programmes includes the components of system change, education, audit and feedback, organisational climate, and infrastructure reminders (WHO, 2016). The latter in the form of "nudging" is receiving increasing traction in IPC. Nudges produce subtle changes to the choice architecture or framing of information that can influence behaviour without restricting choice. A scoping review by Schiller et al. (2020) into nudges and IPC advised they can have a positive impact on IPC and gave examples around hand hygiene compliance, disinfection of equipment and guideline adherence.

The audit and timely feedback of health care practices to relevant staff is core component 6. Audits are posited to increase accountability and improve the quality of hospital care through systematic monitoring and evaluation. The Health and Social Act (2008), a Code of Practice for the Prevention and Control of Infections, outlines a plethora of policies which it states should be monitored and subject to a rolling programme of audit. These include Hand Hygiene and Antimicrobial Stewardship. However, too often audit can become a routine 'monitoring tool' that is not explicitly linked to driving improvement (Wilson, 2018). Audit reports can often engender spurious results of 100% compliance. This probably reveals a tension between conducting an authentic audit, a duty of candour, and reactions that may come from external scrutiny. The success of an audit is shaped by its context and the way it is implemented. Challenges in relation to digital innovation to improve this area of practice are discussed in more detail later.

Core component 7 emphasises the importance of bed occupancy and the workload of healthcare workers. According to the National Audit Office (2018) hospitals work more safely and effectively at occupancy rates no higher than 85%. However, Trusts routinely exceed this figure due to a secular decline in beds and a growing demand for hospital services. Component 7 is closely aligned with Component 8, which recognises that patients should be cared for a clean and hygienic environment and that staff have the material resources to facilitate good infection control practice. The rationale for both components 7 and 8 is that extrinsic risk factors for HCAI include areas such as, hospitalisation, extended stays, high occupancy rates, overcrowding, staff workload, skill mix, mixing patient populations, lack of single rooms, and other equipment (Stewart et al., 2021). In short, avoiding admission and discharging at the earliest opportunity are two sound strategies for avoiding a HCAI. This issue is discussed in more detail later.

Digital innovations in IPC

The integration of digital technology into infection prevention and control (IPC) marks a pivotal evolution in healthcare practices, particularly for nursing. Digital innovations in IPC, ranging from digital monitoring systems that aim to enhance hand hygiene compliance to telehealth platforms reducing the need for in-person visits, represent significant efforts in combating infection risks efficiently and effectively. Exploring the integration of digital technologies into IPC provides valuable insights into the necessity for nurses to be digitally literate, critically assess the utility of new tools, and advocate for technologies that genuinely improve patient care.

The exploration of both successful and less successful digital innovations is vital to understand the process and the roles nurses may play within it. This may ensure that IPC strategies remain effective in the face of rapidly evolving healthcare challenges such as global ageing and increasing multi-morbidity. Crucially, digital innovation is not merely about adopting new technologies but about fostering a culture of innovation, critical thinking, and adaptability within nursing, driving forward the mission of safer, high-quality patient care in the digital age. Whilst some digital technologies may be said to be merely 'disruptive' in that they challenge existing ways of practising nursing, others may be more accurately described as 'transformative' in that they necessitate a more fundamental re-evaluation of the role nurses might play to achieve the same broad aim. This is best illustrated in the context of infection control in online/virtual spaces which represents an entirely new environment within which nursing might be practised clinically. This is considerably different to the physical environment, the cleanliness and safety of which has long been considered a core focus of nursing since the pioneering work of Nightingale on sanitation in the late 19th century.

The following section provides discussion of two key examples of digital innovation in the context of infection control. The first case explores an example of innovation in nursing practices which is yet to be fully realised, based on the growing significance of online and virtual spaces as a new environment within which nursing is practised. The use of telehealth and virtual spaces to provide nursing care is typically looked at from the perspective of increasing access to services or reducing costs. A new perspective is provided here, considering the potentially unique *nursing* perspective and purpose for using such spaces.

The second case explores a (so far) ineffective innovation which highlights the significance of human factors and human-infrastructure in the development and implementation of new technologies. This is explored in the context of a specific clinical activity. Namely, hand hygiene, arguably one of the most important activities nurses perform (and encourage in others) to prevent the spread of communicable disease.

Telehealth and virtual spaces in infection control

The COVID-19 pandemic significantly affected both healthcare systems and society at large, leading to a swift shift towards telehealth as a primary mode of delivering healthcare services (Wosik et al., 2020). Telehealth, which encompasses remote care delivery using devices like laptops, tablets, smartphones, or wearables, enables patients to receive care from healthcare providers or virtual assistants remotely. This shift, though initially prompted by the urgent needs arising from the pandemic, has broader implications for reducing the risk of communicable diseases in healthcare settings. Facilities for inpatient care have historically been associated with the risk of healthcare-acquired infections (HCAIs) and the challenge of antimicrobial resistant (AMR) organism colonisation, which poses a significant threat to global health due to antimicrobial resistance, as discussed by Haque et al. (2018). These risks are reflected in component 8 of the WHO core components of IPC.

Remote care delivery through digital platforms, such as virtual clinics or smartphone apps, offers a strategy to mitigate the risks of infection and AMR organism colonisation. In Italy, for example, a study by Ceradini et al. (2017) demonstrated that virtual collaboration among communicable disease specialists in managing complex cases led to more judicious antibiotic use, a decrease in hospital-acquired infections in critical care settings, fewer instances of multi-drug-resistant organism isolation, and reduced antibiotic expenditures. This study also pointed out the educational advantages for clinicians participating in virtual meetings, though it was limited by its small scale and lack of detail on the composition of the multidisciplinary teams, especially the involvement of nurses in these telemedicine clinics. The evidence from Italy suggests potential benefits, but it remains to be seen how widely these practices are adopted in other contexts like the UK, where the role of nurses in virtual healthcare delivery is still evolving. Nurses should explore the possibilities that virtual healthcare models offer for the specific purpose of preventing HCAIs and managing AMR-related risks.

In the context of nursing practices in online and virtual spaces, the traditional nursing metaparadigm concept of 'environment' (Fawcett, 1984) has been augmented. Modern nurses are required to consider the impacts of a physical environment consisting of real people, real threats such as poor housing, climate change, endemic disease and socially mediated health behaviours. They must also now consider the less tangible digital environment within which patients exist. Including the potential influences of this environment on both salutogenesis and pathogenesis. This shift in the nature of the nursing environment to virtual environments inevitably necessitates consideration of new forms of risk and new interventions to limit the transmission of infection. Whilst in the physical environment, cleaning, ventilation and physical placement of infected or vulnerable individuals in side-wards or bays to limit transmission are now long established in practice and policy, there remains little consideration of how nurses might act in virtual spaces to limit the spread of infection. The new digital environments within which patients exist and engage in information exchange either with health professionals including nurses, or with other people online present new challenges in relation to the control of communicable disease. The internet has facilitated the proliferation of both high- and low-quality information, the consumption of which is compounded by algorithm-driven influences on users' exposure to new information. Reducing trust in newer forms of media (i.e., social media) which is much less regulated than traditional forms of media has been associated with the trend towards declining acceptance and uptake of vaccinations in the post COVID-19 pandemic period (Altman et al., 2023) (see Chapter 4 for more detailed discussion on social media and its impact on nursing). It is evident however, that attention to online/virtual environments (e.g., the metaverse) and how information is disseminated and interpreted in these environments represents an entirely new context for IPC practice which is currently absent from the WHO core components. It stands to reason, given the environment being a metaparadigm concept of nursing that IPC in this area will, and should, become a new focus for nursing practices.

In response to growing demands on conventional healthcare services, there is also growing interest in the concept of 'virtual wards' within which patients receive in-patient care but from home, this is facilitated by remote monitoring systems in addition to traditional in-person care (Norman et al. 2023). However, the evidence underpinning these models is still in its infancy and typically does not consider a reduction in communicable disease transmission as a core purpose of such care models, despite AMR, in particular, being a focus of significant strategic priority in healthcare globally. The benefits of these approaches to 'inpatient' care, however, are obvious in relation to communicable disease transmission. If individuals can receive, for example, their post-surgical care in their own home instead of a highly contaminated surgical ward staffed by clinicians interacting with many other patients in a single shift the risks of infection are likely much reduced. Images illustrating of a user interface for a 'virtual' ward are provided in Figures 6.1.

Applying the Lens for Digital Nursing (LDN) to IPC

To understand how nursing practice might change in relation to the use of virtual spaces and telemedicine in the digital age, a synthesis of key issues is provided below. Utilising the Lens for Digital Nursing (LDN) (see Chapter 1), a synthesis of contemporary nursing theory related to the use of digital technologies (Wynn et al., 2023a, 2023b), the roles of nurses in relation to IPC in online/virtual spaces can be seen in Table 6.2.

As can be seen in Table 6.3. By considering theoretical concepts in nursing such as those within the LDN, potentially new practices of nurses may emerge. For example, at an individual level it is suggested that nurses may engage in IPC practice by discussing the use of online information sources directly with patients to understand where their information comes from and how they interpret it. This is not currently standard practice in nursing and there remain no clear frameworks for how such a practice may be conducted systematically and effectively. In considering the agency of technologies in influencing human behaviour it is suggested that there may be a role for nurses in actively monitoring and understanding the

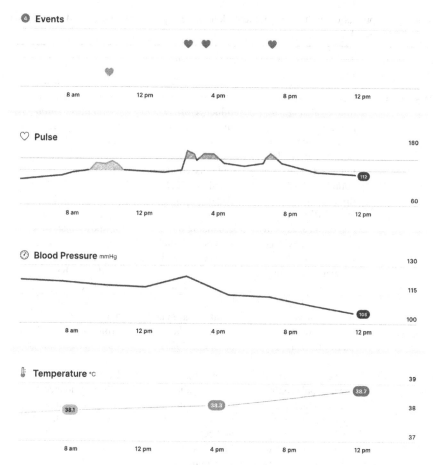

FIGURE 6.1   Virtual ward interface illustrating trends in physiological parameters for a patient over time. Image provided courtesy of **doccla**.

roles that social media algorithms may play in influencing human behaviour associated with communicable disease. Whilst it is currently common for IPC nurses to counsel individual patients on suggested behaviours, for example, self-isolation or cleansing using special products, little attention is paid to the broader influences on human behaviour which are exerted digitally via online spaces.

This theoretical reappraisal of nursing activity based on the associations between digital technology and communicable disease transmission may reflect the need for transformative changes in IPC nursing practice. As previously noted, the requirements of core component 1 of the WHO international guidelines have so far been met with wide variations in team structures and service delivery models. It is arguably therefore feasible that new nursing roles may be developed to reflect the influence of digital technologies in practice. These roles would reflect innovation

TABLE 6.2 Application of the LDN framework to nursing practice in the context of infection control

Level of Practice	Concept – Knowing the Person	Concept – Technology as Agent	Concept – Technological Competency
Population	Awareness of the use of natural language processing and social media data to understand trends in the spread of communicable diseases (Pilipiec et al., 2023) Using online spaces to maintain knowledge of clinical evidence, for example following organisations, journals or healthcare professionals on social media platforms (Davis, 2023)	Recognising the influence of misinformation on patients and the public and its rapid dissemination in online spaces (Vosoughi et al., 2018) Recognising the effects of digital inequalities and their influence patients' digital literacy and access to information and services (Blank and Reisdorf, 2023)	Curating accurate and useful information related to the control of communicable disease (Davis, 2023) Using online interprofessional collaboration to facilitate the sharing of knowledge, best practice and relevant resources Considering the principles of digital professionalism and guidance from professional regulators. For example, the (UK) Nursing and Midwifery Council's (2023) guidance on using social media responsibly should be read in conjunction with the Code
Community	Gaining insight into the local population's health concerns by being active on social media using a professional account (Gisondi et al., 2022) Recognising the role of online communities in influencing health outcomes for patients with long-term communicable diseases (Cao et al., 2017)	Recognising how social media platforms influence disease control and behaviours in different communities (Sooknanan and Comissiong, 2020)	
Individual	Communicating with patients to understand their use of online spaces including how they access and use information from online sources (Gisondi et al., 2022)		Developing competencies in the use of telehealth technology to minimise avoidable in-person care, reducing the risk of healthcare-associated infections and antimicrobial resistance (Ceradini et al., 2017; Wosik et al., 2020)

Adapted from Wynn (2024).

in IPC beyond the plain digitalisation of existing practice, i.e., in the case of hand hygiene monitoring. Examples of these new roles might include *Digital Health Advocates* focussed on enhancing patients' digital health literacy, guiding them through reliable online health information and advocating for digital inclusivity. *Online Community Managers* managing virtual health communities, ensuring the dissemination of accurate information, moderating discussions, and providing support to patients. There is already a growing body of evidence indicating the value of intervention in virtual communities in the context of HIV care, where online spaces have been utilised in environments where potential patients (i.e., dating apps such as Grindr) may already be present to share information and promote self-testing (Cao et al., 2017). Finally, *Telehealth Specialists,* dedicated to identifying patients suitable for remote care delivery and supporting services to operate remotely for the specific purpose of infection control, for example, by specifically seeking to virtualise the care of particularly high-risk patients. Lastly, *Nursing Data Analysts* who combine expertise in data analytics with expert knowledge in IPC to interpret trends from social media and other digital sources, thereby informing and shaping public health and IPC strategies and interventions.

Digital hand hygiene monitoring

Hand hygiene stands as a cornerstone of infection prevention and control (IPC) practices within healthcare settings. Its significance is rooted in historical practices, tracing back to the pioneering work of Ignaz Semmelweis in the mid-19th century. Semmelweis's discovery that hand disinfection could drastically reduce the incidence of puerperal fever revolutionised the approach to patient care and infection control. This fundamental principle of hand hygiene has remained unchanged; however, the methods of ensuring compliance and monitoring have evolved significantly, especially with the advent of digital technology. As discussed earlier, hand hygiene features prominently in components 5 and 6 of the WHO's core components of IPC. Recent years have seen the testing and implementation of various digital hand hygiene monitoring systems. These range from simple badge-based systems, which track the use of hand sanitiser dispensers, to more sophisticated sensor networks that monitor hand washing frequency and technique against established compliance benchmarks. Such systems aim to provide an objective and continuous assessment of hand hygiene practices, moving beyond the limitations of direct observation, typically recorded in hand hygiene audits, which can be labour-intensive and subject to observer bias (Wang et al., 2021).

Despite the critical importance of hand hygiene, adherence to policies based on human factors remains a challenge. Factors such as workload, access to hand hygiene resources, staff attitudes, and the prevailing culture within healthcare institutions can significantly impact compliance rates. Crucially, it has been acknowledged that there is distance between policy makers, who are typically senior clinicians (i.e., IPC nurses) and those who have to enact the policies in frontline care roles, such as ward nurses (Cole, 2015). This distance may contribute towards expectations of practice which are entirely at odds with the realities of clinical practice which in some cases may require nurses and other clinicians to wash their hands with extreme frequency. This cognitive distance between policy and practice is also reflected in somewhat authoritarian language often used within hand hygiene policies indicating that nurses 'must' follow an unrealistic policy (Cole, 2015). This conflicted basis from which digital innovation might occur, building on a pre-existing tension between the expectations of specialist IPC nurses, unrealistic policies and the realities of clinical practice are useful to illustrate how digital innovation in nursing may be undermined. Specifically, digital technologies which seek to enforce existing non-feasible practices are likely doomed to fail to achieve their purpose.

The digital monitoring of nurses and other health professionals' hand hygiene practices introduces a set of implications that extend beyond mere compliance. On the one hand, it offers the potential for targeted interventions, personalised feedback, and a comprehensive understanding of hand hygiene behaviours within clinical settings. On the other hand, it raises questions about privacy, the potential for increased pressure on healthcare workers, and the risk of fostering a culture of surveillance rather than one of support and improvement. In a review by Wang et al. (2021), issues were identified with these technologies which can be seen in Table 6.3.

TABLE 6.3 Challenges identified with digital hand hygiene monitoring

System Accuracy: Variability in metrics, affected by technical issues and geometric constraints, undermines the accuracy of monitoring systems. Hardware limitations and algorithm inaccuracies contribute to the difficulty in reliably tracking hand hygiene compliance and quality.

Data Integration: Integrating data from diverse sensors presents challenges, including calibration discrepancies and data format inconsistencies. These issues complicate the accurate interpretation of hand hygiene behaviours.

Privacy and Confidentiality: Digital monitoring raises concerns about privacy for healthcare workers (HCWs) and patients, potentially viewed as intrusive surveillance, leading to resistance and legal complexities, particularly where cameras are used to track compliance.

Potential Risks: Risks include UV-related harm from monitoring equipment, contamination from wearable devices, infection risks during system installation, and interference with medical devices due to radio-frequency emissions.

Usability: Systems may disrupt HCW's workflows or require behaviour changes for accurate monitoring, with issues like device bulkiness and battery limitations affecting usability.

Associated Costs and Infrastructure: High costs for installation, maintenance, and necessary infrastructure improvements present significant barriers, especially in community healthcare settings.

Performance Feedback: Designing effective, acceptable feedback mechanisms to improve hand hygiene practices without causing anxiety or resistance among HCW's is a challenge.

The apprehensions of healthcare professionals, particularly regarding performance and privacy, underscore the critical role of human factors in the development and deployment of innovative technologies within nursing. A comprehensive review by Wynn et al. (2023a, 2023b) examined demographic variables, such as age, gender, voluntariness of use, and experience, based on the Unified Theory of Acceptance and Use of Technology (UTAUT) (Venkatesh et al., 2003). This analysis revealed how these factors might affect nurses' willingness and ability to embrace technology. The review identified a notable gap in evidence concerning nurses' experiences with digital technology and its impact on their acceptance. Furthermore, the forced introduction of technology was found to potentially hinder acceptance. Notably, the study highlighted the critical importance of technology's usability, particularly among female users, who typically prioritise this over mere functionality, unlike their male counterparts. Given the predominance of women in nursing, this distinction underscores the necessity for careful consideration by those implementing digital technologies.

Digital hand hygiene monitoring systems serve as a prime example of the challenges faced. Their limited use is likely driven by a combination of factors: the impracticality of the policies they are based on, as pointed out by Cole (2015); the systems' poor usability, especially significant in the predominantly female nursing workforce (Wynn et al., 2023a, 2023b); and their likely involuntary introduction, which often occurs without meaningful input from frontline nurses, reflecting the top-down nature of the policies they aim to enforce. This issue, in particular, is somewhat unique within the nursing profession whereby policy makers, typically senior nurses, are often no longer practising clinically (i.e., caring for patients directly). This is in contrast to other health professions such medicine where consultants will continue to work in front line roles and lead clinical teams. This distance and detachment of nursing practices from its human focus as mediated via technology was explored by Rubeis (2023) via the concept of 'adiaphorisation'. Adiaphorisation in nursing refers to the process of detaching nursing actions and decisions, including the use of digital technologies, from their ethical and moral implications. This concept becomes particularly relevant in the context of digital hand hygiene monitoring, as it highlights the cognitive and ethical distance between senior policymakers and frontline nursing staff. Senior policy makers, often removed from the day-to-day realities of clinical practice, may advocate for the implementation of digital monitoring technologies based on their potential to improve compliance and patient outcomes. However, this top-down approach can lead to the adiaphorisation of hand hygiene practices, where the focus shifts from the ethical dimensions of nursing care, such as patient dignity, privacy, and professional autonomy, to the instrumental value of compliance metrics.

The implications of this detachment are multifaceted. First, it risks transforming hand hygiene from an ethical commitment to patient safety into a mechanistic task primarily aimed at fulfilling institutional metrics. This shift not only undermines the professional judgement and autonomy of nurses but also diminishes the relational aspect of care that is central to nursing ethics. Furthermore, the pervasive nature of digital surveillance may contribute to a culture of mistrust, where nurses feel monitored and evaluated by impersonal systems rather than supported by their institutions and colleagues. This environment could potentially erode the intrinsic motivation of healthcare workers to engage in hand hygiene practices, instead fostering compliance driven by surveillance and fear of repercussions.

The evolution of hand hygiene practices from the foundational insights of Ignaz Semmelweis to contemporary digital monitoring systems underscores the complex interplay between innovation and the practical realities of healthcare. While digital technologies offer the promise of enhancing infection prevention through objective and continuous assessment, they also introduce significant challenges, including privacy concerns, the potential for increased pressure on healthcare workers, and the risk of engendering a culture of surveillance. These issues reflect broader implications for the use of digital technology in healthcare: the necessity of balancing technological advancement with ethical considerations, user privacy, and the practicalities of clinical workflows. The case of hand hygiene monitoring reveals the critical need for sensitive implementation strategies that acknowledge the human factors in healthcare settings and existing tensions within the human infrastructure providing the background to ongoing digital innovations. This highlights that successful digital innovation must navigate the fine line between improving care and respecting the rights and realities of those it aims to benefit. At the time of writing, there remains no compelling evidence that automated hand-hygiene monitoring systems are associated with reductions in infection or improved hand hygiene compliance (Gould et al., 2024).

Chapter summary

The progression of infection prevention and control (IPC) from its historical roots to the integration of digital innovations marks a significant transformation in healthcare, emphasising the critical role of nursing in this evolving landscape. As we have seen, the challenges inherent in IPC, including antimicrobial resistance (AMR), resource limitations, and global health crises like pandemics, remain daunting. Yet, the digital innovations in IPC present promising avenues for overcoming these obstacles, provided they are navigated with care and an understanding of their implications.

The exploration of digital hand hygiene monitoring systems and the shift towards telehealth and online/virtual spaces for infection control showcases the dual-edged nature of technological advancements. While these innovations offer potential for enhancing IPC measures and expanding the scope of nursing practice, they also bring forth challenges such as privacy concerns, the risk of surveillance cultures, and the necessity for digital literacy among nurses. The discussion on the importance of human factors and the integration of technology into healthcare underscores the complexity of implementing digital innovations effectively. Nurses, at the heart of IPC efforts, must be equipped with the skills and knowledge to navigate this digital landscape. This requires a commitment to continuous education, a willingness to adapt, and an advocacy for the ethical use of technology that genuinely enhances patient care without compromising privacy or personal interaction. Critically, reflection on existing practices in healthcare is needed to ensure that efforts to digitalise care practices do not inadvertently perpetuate the flaws in healthcare policies which have been the subject of significant critique even in a pre-digital context.

Moreover, the concept of 'environment' in nursing practice is expanding beyond physical spaces to include digital and virtual realms. This shift necessitates a broader understanding of care that encompasses digital literacy, the management of online misinformation, and the fostering of healthy digital communities. The role of nurses is evolving, with a growing responsibility to guide patients and the public through the complexities of health information online and other virtual spaces, ensuring that digital spaces contribute positively to public health outcomes.

In moving forward, the integration of digital innovations into IPC must be approached with a critical eye, balancing the benefits against potential drawbacks. Collaboration across disciplines, thoughtful policy development, and a focus on patient-centred care will be key to navigating the future.

References

Alhumaid, S., Mutair, A., Al Alawi, Z., et al. (2021). Knowledge of infection prevention and control among healthcare workers and factors influencing compliance: A systematic review. *Antimicrobial Resistance & Infection Control, 10*(1), 86. https://doi.org/10.1186/s13756-021-00957-0

Altman, J. D., Miner, D. S., Lee, A. A., Asay, A. E., Nielson, B. U., Rose, A. M., Hinton, K., & Poole, B. D. (2023). Factors affecting vaccine attitudes influenced by the COVID-19 pandemic. *Vaccines, 11*(3), 516. https://doi.org/10.3390/vaccines11030516

Blank, G., & Reisdorf, B. (2023). Digital inequalities and public health during COVID-19: Media dependency and vaccination. *Information, Communication & Society, 26*(5), 1045–1065. https://doi.org/10.1080/1369118X.2023.2166356

Brewster, L., Tarrant, C., & Dixon-Woods, M. (2016). Qualitative study of views and experiences of performance management of healthcare-associated infections. *Journal of Hospital Infection, 41*, 47.

Bynum, B. (2001). Hospitalism. *The Lancet, 357*, 1372.

Cao, B., Gupta, S., Wang, J., et al. (2017). Social media interventions to promote HIV testing, linkage, adherence, and retention: Systematic review and meta-analysis. *Journal of Medical Internet Research, 19*(11), e394. https://doi.org/10.2196/jmir.7997

Centers for Disease Control and Prevention. (2001). Updated guidelines for evaluating public health surveillance systems: Recommendations from the guidelines working group. *MMWR Recommendations and Reports, 50*, 1–35.

Centre for Workforce Intelligence. (2015). *Review of the infection prevention and control nurse workforce.* CFWI, London.

Ceradini, J., Tozzi, A. E., D'Argenio, P., et al. (2017). Telemedicine as an effective intervention to improve antibiotic appropriateness prescription and to reduce costs in pediatrics. *Italian Journal of Pediatrics, 43*(1), 105. https://doi.org/10.1186/s13052-017-0423-3

Cole, M. (2015). A discourse analysis of hand hygiene policy in NHS Trusts. *Journal of Infection Prevention, 16*(4), 156–161. https://doi.org/10.1177/1757177415575412

Davis, D. (2023). Digital curation: Implications for the nursing student and nursing practice. In Vasilica, C. M., Gillaspy, E., & Withnell, N. (Eds.), *Digital skills for nursing studies and practice* (pp. 85–99). Learning Matters, London.

Fawcett, J. (1984). The metaparadigm of nursing: Present status and future refinements. *Image: The Journal of Nursing Scholarship, 16*(3), 84–87. https://doi.org/10.1111/j.1547-5069.1984.tb01393.x

Gisondi, M. A., Barber, R., Faust, J. S., et al. (2022). A deadly infodemic: Social media and the power of COVID-19 misinformation. *Journal of Medical Internet Research, 24*(2), e35552. https://doi.org/10.2196/35552

Gould, D., Hawker, C., Drey, N., & Purssell, E. (2024). Should automated electronic hand-hygiene monitoring systems be implemented in routine patient care? Systematic review and appraisal with Medical Research Council Framework for Complex Interventions. *Journal of Hospital Infection, 147*, 180–187. https://doi.org/10.1016/j.jhin.2024.03.012

Guest, J. F., Keating, T., Gould, D., et al. (2020). Modelling the annual NHS costs and outcomes attributable to healthcare-associated infections in England. *BMJ Open, 10*, e033367. https://doi.org/10.1136/bmjopen-2019-033367

Haley, R. W., Culver, D. H., White, J. W., Morgan, W. M., Emori, T. G., Munn, V. P., & Hooton, T. M. (1985). The efficacy of infection surveillance and control programs in preventing nosocomial infections in US hospitals. *American Journal of Epidemiology, 121*(2), 182–205. https://doi.org/10.1093/oxfordjournals.aje.a113990

Haque, M., Sartelli, M., McKimm, J., & Abu Bakar, M. (2018). Health care-associated infections – An overview. *Infection and Drug Resistance, 11*, 2321–2333. https://doi.org/10.2147/IDR.S177247

Health and Social Care Act. (2008). *A code of practice on the prevention and control of infections.* Crown Copyright. Retrieved from https://www.gov.uk/government/publications/the-health-and-social-care-act-2008-code-of-practice-on-the-prevention-and-control-of-infections-and-related-guidance/health-and-social-care-act-2008-code-of-practice-on-the-prevention-and-control-of-infections-and-related-guidance

Knight, G., Pham, T., Stimson, J., et al. (2022). The contribution of hospital-acquired infections to the COVID-19 epidemic in England in the first half of 2020. *BMC Infectious Diseases, 22*(1), 556.

Lavellee, J., Gray, T., Dumville, J., et al. (2017). The effects of bundles on patient outcomes: A systematic review and meta-analysis. *Implementation Science, 12*, 142.

Michaleas, S., Laios, K., Charalabopoulos, A., et al. (2022). Joseph Lister (1827–1912): A pioneer of antiseptic surgery. *Cureus, 14*(12). https://doi.org/10.7759/cureus.32777

Mitchell, B., Fasugba, O., & Russo, P. (2020). Where is the strength of the evidence? A review of infection prevention and control guidelines. *Journal of Hospital Infection, 105*(2), 242–251. https://doi.org/10.1016/j.jhin.2020.01.008

National Audit Office. (2018). *Report by the comptroller and auditor general: Reducing emergency admissions.* Department of Health & Social Care, NHS England.

Norman, G., Bennett, P., & Vardy, E. R. L. C. (2023). Virtual wards: A rapid evidence synthesis and implications for the care of older people. *Age and Ageing, 52*(1), afac319. https://doi.org/10.1093/ageing/afac319

Nursing and Midwifery Council. (2023). Social media guidance. Retrieved from https://www.nmc.org.uk/standards/guidance/social-media-guidance

Pereira, V., Silva, S., Carvalho, V., et al. (2022). Strategies for the implementation of clinical practice guidelines in public health: An overview of systematic reviews. *Health, 20*(1), 13. https://doi.org/10.1186/s12961-022-00815-4

Perry, C. (2005). The infection control nurse in England – Past, present, and future. *British Journal of Infection Control, 6*(5), 18–21.

Pilipiec, P., Samsten, I., & Bota, A. (2023). Surveillance of communicable diseases using social media: A systematic review. *PLoS One, 18*(2), e0282101. https://doi.org/10.1371/journal.pone.0282101

Ridelberg, M., & Nilsen, P. (2015). Using surveillance data to reduce healthcare-associated infection: A qualitative study in Sweden. *Journal of Infection Prevention, 16*(5), 208–214. https://doi.org/10.1177/1757177415588380

Rubeis, G. (2023). Adiaphorisation and the digital nursing gaze: Liquid surveillance in long-term care. *Nursing Philosophy, 24*, e12388. https://doi.org/10.1111/nup.12388

Schiller, S., Bludau, A., Mathes, T., et al. (2020). Unpacking nudge sensu lato: Insights from a scoping review. *Journal of Hospital Infection, 143*, 168–177. https://doi.org/10.1016/j.jhin.2023.11.001

Smith, P., Watkins, K., & Hewlett, A. (2011). Infection control through the ages. *American Journal of Infection Control, 40*, 35–42.

Sooknanan, J., & Comissiong, D. M. (2020). Trending on social media: Integrating social media into infectious disease dynamics. *Bulletin of Mathematical Biology, 82*(7), 86. https://doi.org/10.1007/s11538-020-00757-4

Stewart, S., Robertson, C., & Pan, J. (2021). Impact of healthcare-associated infection on length of stay. *Journal of Hospital Infection, 114*, 23–31. https://doi.org/10.1016/j.jhin.2021.02.026

UK Health Security Agency. (2023). *Annual epidemiological commentary, up to and including financial year April 2022 to March 2023.* Crown Copyright. Retrieved from https://www.gov.uk/government/statistics/mrsa-mssa-and-e-coli-bacteraemia-and-c-difficile-infection-annual-epidemiological-commentary/annual-epidemiological-commentary-gram-negative-mrsa-mssa-bacteraemia-and-c-difficile-infections-up-to-and-including-financial-year-2022-to-2023#:~:text=During%20the%20financial%20year%20(%20FY,remaining%20below%20pre%2Dpandemic%20levels.

Venkatesh, V., Morris, M. G., Davis, F. D., & Davis, G. B. (2003). User acceptance of information technology: Toward a unified view. *MIS Quarterly, 27*, 425–478.

Vosoughi, S., Roy, D., & Aral, S. (2018). The spread of true and false news online. *Science, 359*(6380), 1146–1151. https://doi.org/10.1126/science.aap9559

Wang, C., Jiang, W., Yang, K., Yu, D., Newn, J., Sarsenbayeva, Z., Goncalves, J., & Kostakos, V. (2021). Electronic monitoring systems for hand hygiene: Systematic review of technology. *Journal of Medical Internet Research, 23*(11), e27880. https://doi.org/10.2196/27880

Wilson J. (2018). Rethinking the use of audit to drive improvement. *Journal of Infection Prevention, 19*(1), 3–4. https://doi.org/10.1177/1757177417746732

Wilson, J. (2019). *Infection control in clinical practice* (3rd ed.). Elsevier, London.

World Health Organisation (WHO). (2011). *Report on the burden of endemic health care-associated infection worldwide.* WHO, Geneva.

World Health Organisation (WHO). (2016). *Guidelines on core components of infection control programmes at the national and acute health care facility level.* WHO, Geneva.

Wosik, J., Fudim, M., Cameron, B., Gellad, Z. F., Cho, A., Phinney, D., Curtis, S., Roman, M., Poon, E. G., Ferranti, J., Katz, J. N., & Tcheng, J. (2020). Telehealth transformation:

COVID-19 and the rise of virtual care. *Journal of the American Medical Informatics Association, 27*(6), 957–962. https://doi.org/10.1093/jamia/ocaa067

Wynn, M., Garwood-Cross, L., Vasilica, C., Griffiths, M., Heaslip, V., & Phillips, N. (2023b). Digitizing nursing: A theoretical and holistic exploration to understand the adoption and use of digital technologies by nurses. *Journal of Advanced Nursing, 79*, 3737–3747. https://doi.org/10.1111/jan.15810

Wynn, M., Garwood-Cross, L., Vasilica, C., & Davis, D. (2023a). Digital nursing practice theory: A scoping review and thematic analysis. *Journal of Advanced Nursing, 79*(11), 4137–4148. https://doi.org/10.1111/jan.15660

Wynn, M. (2024). Online spaces and the control of communicable diseases: Implications for nursing practice. *Nursing Standard.* https://doi.org/10.7748/ns.2024.e12174

7

THE FUTURE OF NURSING

Louise Cave and Gillian Strudwick

A vision for the future

Anticipating the future of nursing in the digital age, this concluding chapter explores emerging technologies and their potential impact on the nursing profession. From robotics to AI and telehealth, readers will discover a visionary landscape of possibilities. Interprofessional collaboration and patient empowerment are discussed, inspiring nurses to be at the forefront of shaping their profession's future in the digital era.

The world is advancing with technology faster than sci-fi writers can keep up with, and we have to stop and ask ourselves: what does this mean for nurses in the future? How will the role change? Where can technology take us? The role of a nurse is changing; the traditional boundaries and competencies of a nurse are expanding. New roles are being introduced that are bridging the healthcare and technology gaps. Nursing leaders are now required to contribute to policies and processes for the future of healthcare delivery. This chapter explores the numerous ways the nursing role is changing through the introduction and development of technologies. As healthcare systems expand to meet the ever-growing populations of the world, nurses will continue to move further away from traditional nursing models of care. Nurses are the largest health and care professional group globally (World Health Organization [WHO], 2020) and, in current practice, are often the ones spending the most time face-to-face with patients (either in person or via a digital device). In the digital age, the future of nursing is poised to be transformative, focusing on interprofessional collaboration, patient empowerment, and nurses taking on further leadership roles in healthcare and the technology sector.

The global population continues to grow, and many countries face an aging population, leading to an increased demand for healthcare services. The number

DOI: 10.4324/9781032714547-7

TABLE 7.1 The global decline in nurses

Year	Global Population (Billions)	Number of Nurses (Millions)	Nurses Per Capita
2000	6.1	28	218
2005	6.5	27	240
2010	6.9	26	265
2015	7.3	24	304
2020	7.8	22	354

Figure 1. Data sources: World Bank, WHO.

of nurses globally is also decreasing. Each year, the World Health Organization (2020) estimates a global shortfall of approximately 6 million nurses. Table 7.1 shows the decline in the number of nurses globally. With the continual shortfall, governments across the globe are looking to technology to meet healthcare system gaps.

The digital revolution is often seen as at odds with the empathetic, caring nature of nursing, with nurses emphasising the importance of their role in providing compassionate, humanised care (Strudwick et al., 2020). Technology is seen to add new hurdles for nurses to overcome when developing the therapeutic relationship. Technology itself tests what we understand by the term "therapeutic relationship", as it moves away from being defined as 'a significant knowing and meaningful connectedness' that involves understanding the patient as a whole person, fostering a strong mutual connection that is protective, trustful, and humanistic (Mirhaghi et al., 2017). Technology will inherently challenge this definition by having a deeper understanding of a patient in an instant, while it may take nurses weeks to develop this with a patient. This has the power to change the therapeutic relationship for the better, but it also has the potential to be filled with various biases.

Nursing theory plays a crucial role in shaping the future of nursing practice, especially in the context of the digital age. Theories related to digital nursing practice emphasise the role of technology as an agent within the patient environment, nurse interactions with technology to achieve 'knowing' of patients, and the necessity of technological competence among nurses (Wynn et al., 2023). Throughout this chapter, we will explore how nursing theories must evolve to incorporate the role of digital technologies in healthcare. Crucially, it is important to continue to consider what it means to be a nurse and what it could mean to be a nurse in the future.

When looking to the future, it is of the utmost importance that nurses use their voices to have a say in where their place is in the future of healthcare delivery. Due to nurses being the largest healthcare group in the workforce, they need to be active stakeholders. They can – and should – inform key technology decisions to ensure sustainability for the future. They must lead the way in researching and adapting their practice to ensure that care delivered by nurses tomorrow is no less valuable than care delivered by nurses today. The growing populations of tomorrow require nurses to work differently and think differently. As nurses, it is our responsibility to think of the future of global health and understand our vital role in ensuring that safe care is delivered in the centuries to come.

What is the future process of nursing?

There is a multitude of research and theories available that attempt to explain the process of nursing; however, theorist Orlando (1961) proposed the model of assessment, diagnosis, planning, implementation, and evaluation which, alongside Roper, Logan, and Tierney's (2000) assessment of activities of daily living model (Figure 7.1), can be used to understand the current state of the nursing process. This model has been focused upon, as it remains widely taught to nursing students globally and encompasses all elements of nursing care. The current focus for healthcare system redesign has been to integrate technology into each stage of the nursing process. Health systems have streamlined data collection and analysis during the assessment phase, ensuring more accurate and timely information. We have begun to see advanced diagnostic tools powered by AI supporting nurses in forming diagnoses. Planning and intervention have been optimised through digital care plans and telehealth services, enabling better coordination and delivery of care. Technology has facilitated continuous evaluation through real-time monitoring and

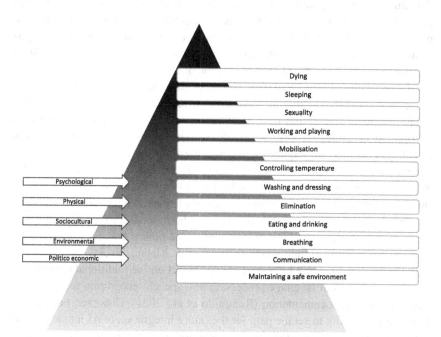

FIGURE 7.1 Roper, Logan, and Tierney model.

feedback systems, ensuring that patient outcomes are consistently reviewed and improved.

We have reached an inflection point, where we have used the current nursing process and models, and in many areas, we have optimised where possible. We must now consider whether the future models of healthcare and the nursing process should indeed follow the historic nursing process models or whether the nursing process of the future must change and adapt to a new theoretical model (Wynn et al., 2023). This is a challenge, however, as the approach to the digitisation of nursing has varied widely. With digital tools operating at diverse levels, there needs to be systematic integration of theory development and social debate (Tischendorf et al., 2024).

This is where we must turn to our nursing leaders to evolve our use of technology and generate new scientific knowledge (Booth et al., 2021). Nurses must look to the future to develop new models of practice. It is not for the technology industry to decide the future models of nursing care; rather, it is for nurses to lead with research, evidence, and future efficiency in mind. Further discussion of the particular issues of how nursing identity and practice are developed is provided in Chapter 1.

The start of the artificial intelligence (AI) revolution

The future of nursing cannot be discussed without first looking towards AI, although it does not have all the answers. Over the last decade, we have seen an increase in the use of AI within healthcare, using machine learning and natural language processing techniques and applying them to healthcare datasets (Booth et al., 2021). This has aided the widespread implementation of electronic health records globally and the recording of structured data. However, this has only furthered the 'digital divide' and associated healthcare inequalities (Shaw, 2023). Within England, there remain hospitals that do not have electronic health records, retaining all patient information on paper records. Standardised nursing language and taxonomy in digital systems are also required to support the future developments of systems. When they are not in place, clinical decision support and care planning are full of challenges (Hants et al., 2023). Nurse leaders play a vital role in ensuring that the foundation blocks of digital technology are implemented into healthcare systems and that future developments can be used and harnessed (Shaw, 2023). We need nurses to take active leadership roles to influence policy decisions, standards of practice, and regulatory frameworks (Strudwick & Risling, 2024).

We have already seen AI demonstrate an impact on the traditional nursing process, by using natural language processing and speech recognition technology to speed up nursing documentation (Ronquillo et al., 2021). However, nurses have shared responsibility to set the path for the future integration of AI into healthcare systems. Nurses should ensure this is ethical and aligns with core nursing values such as compassionate care (Buchanan et al., 2020). Though to do this, nurses must be clear and rigorous on what the core values of the profession are. Schmidt and McArthur (2018) explore the lack of clarity in nursing values and provide the following definition:

> Professional nursing values are defined as important professional nursing principles of human dignity, integrity, altruism, and justice that serve as a framework for standards, professional practice, and evaluation.
>
> *(Schmidt & McArthur, 2018, p. 72)*

Generative Artificial Intelligence is an area of technology where we cannot even begin to predict the learning. Generative AI is a technology that can create new data, such as text and images, based on existing input. In nursing care, it is applied to reduce nurses' repetitive electronic documentation tasks by automating the creation of nursing records. This technology has the potential to ease the workload of nurses by generating accurate and comprehensive nursing records, including structured assessments and narrative records, based on virtual patient data (Lee et al., 2024). AI is currently being used in healthcare to better understand large datasets, however, the more we use this to understand the many variables associated with an individual's health management, the more gaps in the research and understanding will be identified.

We have recently seen the introduction of ChatGPT, developed by OpenAI, which was introduced to the general public in November 2022. This marked the launch of a user-friendly interface for interacting with the language model, enabling widespread access and use. However, this meant that we saw some of the first cases of healthcare professionals exploring the use of ChatGPT to inform their care delivery and planning (Ayoub et al., 2023). This has raised many issues around the accuracy, reliability, privacy, and security of the tool for healthcare. All future implementations of generative AI within healthcare require careful planning, execution, and management of expectations, with a focus on factors such as data privacy, security, and the irreplaceable role of clinicians' expertise (Reddy, 2024).

Clinical decision support

The integration of Artificial Intelligence in clinical decision support (CDS) systems is poised to revolutionise nursing practice. This transformation is driven by AI's ability to enhance decision-making, improve patient outcomes, and streamline clinical workflows. AI and machine learning models are evolving to support clinical decision-making in complex care scenarios. For instance, AI can assist in monitoring cardiovascular patients in intensive care units (ICUs) by analysing clinical time series and electronic health records data, using methods like gradient boosting and recurrent neural networks (Moazemi et al., 2023). We must begin to look to the future of nursing, such as recognising tasks that do not add immediate value to patient care and that present an opportunity for partial or full delegation to AI by nurses, which must be done in accordance with research and evidence (Booth et al., 2021). CDS is an example of AI taking on elements of the person's physical health monitoring that the nurse cannot do.

CDS systems can be used to analyse the vast amounts of data given to nurses, which at present cannot adequately be processed during in-the-moment decision points (Strudwick & Risling, 2024). CDS will ensure the most informed decisions are made at any point in time. CDS systems play a crucial role in supporting nurses with tasks such as medication management, dosage calculation, and care planning. For example, these systems can identify and alert nurses to potential drug interactions, recommend appropriate interventions informed by a patient's medical history and current condition, and provide robust decision support in complex clinical scenarios. The integration of CDSs into nursing practice enhances the precision and safety of patient care, mitigating the risk of medication errors and ensuring that clinical interventions are more accurately tailored to the patient's unique needs, thereby contributing to improved health outcomes.

When looking at the compassionate care model of nursing (Gharouifard et al., 2022), many argue that technology has limited value to the palliative care nursing model, due to the model's ultimate emphasis on the development of the therapeutic relationship between nurse and patient (Dobrina et al., 2014). However, much of the research into the negative effect of technology on the nurse and patient therapeutic relationship is dated and does not account for the advancements made over the past decade. Recent research has shown that AI tools can support palliative care clinicians by predicting short-term mortality risk, complications, and the need for supportive care services, thereby improving decision-making and reducing manual workload (Reddy et al., 2023). This is an example of AI beginning to develop predictive tools that can support elements that are often seen as the art of nursing and not the science. If AI can be shown to make an impact in an area that is seen as the art of nursing, this brings us back to the question of *what does it mean to receive nursing care?*

AI also introduces risks, such as perpetuating human biases, exemplified by a clinical algorithm that prioritised less sick white patients over sicker Black patients in the US (Ronquillo et al., 2021). There is a concern that AI could drive efficiency over quality, reallocating freed-up time towards increased patient volume rather than enhancing care quality (Ronquillo et al., 2021). However, this also identifies a key area for the future roles of nurses in working with AI developers to ensure that the datasets used to build models do not contain unconscious bias. Nurses are best placed to explain the current nuances and anomalies in the data, but they do require further education and training to do this (O'Connor et al., 2023).

Personalised care planning

The future of nursing will see us move to truly personalised models of care. A patient portal and a care plan for both acute and chronic conditions will be available, and patients' health data will no longer be guarded behind paper and unintegrated electronic health records. Personalised care plans will be synced to all devices. We will be able to use AI to predict clinical outcomes, such as short-term mortality risk or survival within six months and forecast the need for supportive care services in cancer patients (Reddy et al., 2023). This will mean that we can provide the right nursing intervention at the right time, rather than inadvertently causing the development of the "sick role". The concept of patients assuming the "sick role" due to over-attentive nursing refers to a phenomenon where excessive care and attention from healthcare providers lead patients to increasingly identify with being ill. This heightened focus on their illness can reinforce dependency and perpetuate behaviours and attitudes consistent with chronic illness, even when the patient's condition does not justify such a stance (Miczo, 2004). This can hinder recovery, reduce motivation to regain independence, and create a cycle of dependency on nursing care.

While there is still limited research into personalised digitalised care planning for physical health, there is an increasing body of evidence from the mental health field (O'Connor et al., 2024). AI technologies in psychiatric nursing are being used to create personalised care plans, monitor symptoms, and assess risks for conditions like dementia, autism, and schizophrenia (Li et al., 2024a, 2024b). This, coupled with a global shift in the acceptance and awareness of mental health conditions, is beginning to enable better multidisciplinary working from healthcare professionals. Nevertheless, the outcomes for individuals with mental health conditions and physical health comorbidities remain poor. There are also limited longitudinal studies on the use of AI in personalised care planning, which would allow for an evaluation of the durability and effectiveness of applications in this area (Li et al., 2024a, 2024b).

Health promotion

Nurses currently use social media extensively for professional development, knowledge sharing, and health promotion across various domains, including sexual and oral health. The COVID-19 pandemic has further underscored the utility of social media in disseminating critical health information and supporting professional networks.

In the future, the potential of social media to scale health promotion efforts and effect sustainable behavioural change is significant. However, addressing challenges such as the digital divide and ensuring robust, evidence-based interventions will be crucial. Specific populations, such as cancer survivors and Indigenous communities, can particularly benefit from well-designed social media health promotion strategies. By leveraging social media and other innovative methods, nurses can continue to play a pivotal role in health promotion, both now and in the future.

We have already seen that AI can aid public health delivery via spatial modelling, risk prediction, misinformation control, public health surveillance, disease forecasting, pandemic/epidemic modelling, and health diagnosis (Olawade et al., 2023). In the future, we can expect to see further research that combines multiple available datasets that now exist due to the digital world, maximising public health surveillance and outbreak control.

Patient empowerment

The future of healthcare should be focused on the democratisation of healthcare data. Personal healthcare data should not be for your clinical team to own and for the individual to request access to. The future of healthcare is freeing health-care data for all, to enable a better-informed general population who understand their health and conditions and who can become much more expert patients. Russo et al. (2019) stress the importance of empowering patients to co-create sustainable healthcare value, emphasising the shift from passive recipients to active stakehold-ers in healthcare decisions. Patient empowerment-focused interventions have been shown to enhance adherence to treatment regimens and reduce healthcare costs (Mogueo & Defo, 2022).

Patient empowerment has been recognised as a measurable outcome for chronic conditions, highlighting the shift towards patient-cantered care and self-manage-ment in healthcare delivery (McAllister et al., 2012). By involving patients in deci-sion-making processes and care plans, healthcare providers can promote autonomy and improve patient outcomes.

With many of the areas discussed, the defined benefit identified is to free up nursing time; however, this is still focused upon the traditional nursing models and theories. The thought is that by leveraging technology, healthcare systems can help alleviate some pressure by improving efficiency and extending the reach of services (Conte et al., 2023). For example, the expectation is that by giving nurses more time, they might be able to either see more patients or deliver a better quality of care to patients in the time they have, with a presumed increased focus upon the patient. However, there are concerns that while AI could drive efficiency, this could reduce overall quality of care delivered. This focus on reallocating freed-up time towards increased patient volume rather than enhancing care quality challenges nursing models like those discussed in Figure 7.1 (Ronquillo et al., 2021). Neither of these disbenefits have yet been demonstrated within the research (Buchanan et al., 2020), although there are preliminary discussions as to what is the intended benefit we want to see with nurses' use of AI.

To ensure positive outcomes, AI development must prioritise *values* that enhance decision-making and remove biases. Nurses must understand AI's development and implications to maintain *ethical* and *effective* practice. This requires a shift in approach to nurse education and requires us to encourage nurses to prioritise career-long learning into technological developments as well as evidence-based research (Rony et al., 2024). Despite AI's potential, critical discourse on its use in nursing is limited, and nursing education struggles to incorporate basic informatics competencies. These issues must be addressed in all future development of AI for healthcare systems. This gap in AI knowledge could exacerbate existing challenges in health informatics, highlighting the need for better integration of AI education in nursing curricula globally.

Robotics

The future of robotics in nursing is poised for significant advancements, driven by technological innovations and the increasing demand for efficient healthcare delivery. Nurses are already using robots within clinical practice to varying degrees in areas such as rehabilitation, pain management, conversation, and education delivery (Buchanan, 2020). Robots within nursing can be looked at in four fundamental areas: assistive robots, social–human-robot interaction, medication delivery, and surgery (Tischendorf et al., 2024).

Assistive robots

Assistive robots are primarily used for physical care tasks such as service delivery and patient monitoring. These robots help in reducing the physical workload on nurses by performing repetitive and physically demanding tasks (Maalouf et al., 2018). Robots are increasingly being used for monitoring patients and alerting healthcare providers about critical changes in patient conditions. This application is crucial in ICUs where continuous monitoring is essential (Li et al., 2024a, 2024b). Robots will also play a valuable role in the community to assist individuals in maintaining their activities of daily living. They will help with medication management and medication delivery. For example, it would be much easier for a drone to deliver your repeat prescription than for a person to do so.

Many studies have suggested that robots help in reducing the workload of nurses by taking over routine tasks, allowing nurses to focus on more critical aspects of patient care (Kangasniemi et al., 2019). Integration of robots in nursing care has been shown to improve overall efficiency in healthcare settings, leading to better resource utilisation and reduced operational costs (Kangasniemi et al., 2019). However, this causes us to return to our nursing models to understand what the critical human-required elements of nursing care are, that cannot be replaced by robots and artificial intelligence. There have been studies that suggest that the current use of robotics within medication adherence can be damaging to the nurse-patient therapeutic relationship (Buchanan, 2020). However, studies into human-robot interaction remain limited, and the consensus is that while there is interest in robots, there is also a very real ambivalence towards them and a lack of comparative research to understand the benefits and disbenefits of robots in healthcare (Zafrani & Nimrod, 2019). Instead of using this as a reason not to implement technology, we must begin to research and understand what the future of the nurse therapeutic relationship should look like when assisted by robotic technology. How can we support and develop better therapeutic relationships for the future? Nurses should be encouraged to imagine the possibilities of what can be actualised through the convergence of AI, robotics, and nursing care (Buchanan, 2020).

Social assistive robots

Earlier in the chapter, we discussed the increasingly aging population and the need to be able to provide healthcare to the masses. Social isolation is a key determinant of health and well-being among the elderly and is often a challenging problem to address due to the workforce needed to address it. The Western modern family home no longer sees elderly relatives live with families until death, as the family is often geographically spread. Social assistive robots focus on the cognitive and emotional well-being of patients, providing companionship and emotional support, particularly for the elderly and those with chronic conditions (Maalouf et al., 2018). This can help to reduce an individual's reliance on the need for nurse support by providing them with the companionship that nurses delivering efficient healthcare do not have the allocated time to provide. There is a growing emphasis on improving human-robot interaction to make these robots more acceptable and effective in providing emotional support (Gibelli et al., 2021).

Is it the case then that we might see a future where human nurses will not be required to deliver the emotional support that is a requisite of so many modern healthcare models? If this is to be the case, continued research on improving human-robot interaction will be crucial in terms of increasing the acceptance and effectiveness of robots in nursing care (Maalouf et al., 2018). Currently, the excessive cost associated with robotic systems and the need for equitable access to these technologies are significant barriers. Efforts are needed to make these technologies more affordable and accessible to a broader population (Servaty et al., 2020). One of the primary ethical concerns is the potential dehumanisation of healthcare due to the increased use of robots. This concern has been exacerbated by the COVID-19 pandemic, which necessitated minimising human contact (Gibelli et al., 2021). As a result, we saw the frustration and technology burnout that can be experienced by many, which needs to be considered when exploring the future of nursing.

Conversely, there have been studies that suggest patients prefer interactions with robots over in-person examinations (Jafari et al., 2022). A review found that cultural factors significantly influence attitudes towards humanoid and animal-like robots. People tend to prefer robots that exhibit behaviours and communication styles aligned with their own culture, suggesting that cultural adaptation is crucial for robot acceptance in healthcare (Papadopoulos & Koulouglioti, 2018). Research exploring the moral judgments made by patients about human and robot interactions found that the moral acceptance was higher with robots, as they respected patient autonomy. However, human interactions were perceived as warmer and more responsible than robots. This brings us back to our nursing theories and the need to evaluate the role of the nurse and the importance and meaning of the therapeutic relationship. Robots are being shown to be acceptable, if not preferred in some instances; therefore, *does a physically present nurse always have to be an essential requirement of nursing?*

Medication delivery and patient safety

Robots are used to deliver medications, ensuring timely and accurate administration, which enhances patient safety and reduces medication errors (Kangasniemi et al., 2019). Robots in this context can be technology that is now commonplace within healthcare systems, such as intravenous smart pumps, or increasingly complex, such as nanobots that have been used for drug delivery.

Nanobots are an emerging field in healthcare, where the role of the nurse might be to monitor a patient as they undergo a procedure performed by nanobots. Nanobots have applications in pain management, where they have been used in both acute and chronic pain management to deliver pain-relieving drugs to the site of pain. They have also been used to diagnose the underlying cause of the pain (Chakravarthy et al., 2018). Nanobots have similarly been used in cancer treatment for targeted drug delivery to specific cells or tissue. This has benefitted patients by reducing side effects and has enhanced the efficacy of chemotherapeutic agents (Brakmane et al., 2012). The concept of Theranostics is also becoming an increasingly researched area with many applications within healthcare; this involves using nanobots for both diagnostic and therapeutic purposes. Nanobots can be used to detect cancerous cells and deliver treatment simultaneously (Kumar et al., 2023; Brakmane et al., 2012).

Hypothetically, when we look towards the future of healthcare, this could mean considerable changes to the role of the nurse. Nurses could be using nanobots to monitor disease progression and aid diagnosis. This could represent a significant change as to how chronic conditions are managed and supported by clinical nurse specialists. Nurses will be required to have the skills and knowledge to educate and support patients. For example, in the COVID-19 pandemic, we saw the rise of conspiracy theories suggesting that Microsoft owner Bill Gates was using the vaccine to microchip the general population. This, and similar conspiracy theories, led to many negative health behaviours; it was spread by both educated professionals (such as doctors) and uneducated individuals (Earnshaw et al., 2020). From this, we can see that there will be educational and ethical hurdles to overcome with the introduction of nanobots to healthcare. With prolific misinformation online, nurses will have to become confident experts, not only to support layperson understanding but also to signpost them to scientific and trusted research (Sharman, 2023).

Surgical robots are already taking healthcare systems by storm globally and are currently still the role of the surgeon to support. However, like many procedures through history, it will not be long before these procedures are performed and led by nurses. When the technology can statistically tell you how safe the procedure will be on the patient, with accuracy, the safety requirement and the need for a highly specialised surgeon to configure and supervise the robot will be minimised. This risk will continue to be assessed by healthcare systems and therefore, in years to come, this could be an expansive area of surgical nursing. The use of robots has been associated with improved patient safety outcomes, including reduced infection rates and fewer medical errors (Kangasniemi et al., 2019). Surgical nurses will have to become experts in the setting up of complex machinery, learn how to work and change the instruments for the robots throughout the surgery. They will be required to develop an intimate technical understanding of the robot, to recognise when it is not working properly and prevent a clinical safety incident. Advances in telesurgery and remote care technologies will enable robots to perform surgical procedures and provide care remotely, expanding access to specialised healthcare services (Jain et al., 2024). This has been purported as a goal of many large tech companies, most recently seen with Microsoft HoloLens and the development of their augmented reality to prepare the public for the future of healthcare.

Remote monitoring

When asked to consider the future of remote monitoring, many will describe virtual wards and the implementation of a centralised data dashboard. However, the reality is that this is the present landscape of nursing in which we find ourselves. The future for remote monitoring will involve drones and targeted interventions delivered by nurses remotely to support the individual (Bhatt et al., 2018). Drones are already being used to help in disaster relief to provide care alongside remote monitoring technology, and they have begun to be used to expedite laboratory testing. Expansion and future research and development in this area could fundamentally change models of care, as unmanned drones in the future could make it much easier to deliver care to patients in the home environment. AI-enabled robotics and telehealth solutions expand the reach of nursing care, improving accessibility and remote monitoring capabilities of patients' health conditions (Rony et al., 2024).

Future approaches to remote monitoring will be multi-faceted, combining many of the technologies previously discussed, coupled with advances in genomic research. Moving forward, it is this combination of technology and scientific research that will disrupt the current nursing models, possibly even to the point of irrelevance.

Visualise, for a moment, the following theoretical scenario: A cancer patient receiving portable intravenous immunotherapy agents experiences a reaction at home. Before the patient fully realises they are reacting, the healthcare professional is already aware, due to the changes in blood cortisol levels, or the patient's observations beginning to worsen. The nurse will be able to react and pause the medication being delivered via their infusion pump, remotely. They will then be able to monitor the impact of this on the disease by looking at a dashboard linked to the nanobot monitoring the tumour site. The nurse will then take this to the multidisciplinary team meeting with the patient's doctor, and the doctor will use AI-assisted genomic medicine to adjust the immunotherapy appropriately.

This may seem a faraway example now; however, in reality, all this relies upon is the convergence of multiple innovative technologies and changes to the current healthcare and nursing models. This changes entirely how we should view nursing models of care, and from this, we can see the many roles that combined technologies may displace nurses from. Nurses must lead the way in how we will use these technologies for the future, as remote monitoring technologies have the power to take care back into the home and reshape the healthcare systems of the future.

Returning once more, to the Roper, Logan, and Tierney (RLT) model, with its focus on the activities of daily living (ADLs), which has long been a cornerstone of nursing practice. Traditionally, this model has relied heavily on direct, physical interactions between nurses and patients, emphasising the importance of human presence in delivering care. However, as the healthcare landscape evolves with the advent of transformative technologies, the application of the RLT model is also poised to undergo significant changes. Table 7.2 illustrates the contrast between

TABLE 7.2 A reflection on potential changes in nursing based on a single popular nursing theory

Activities of Daily Living (ADLs) from RLT Model	Contemporary (Non-Digital) Application	Radical Digital/Technological Transformation
Maintaining a safe environment	Nurses assess and ensure patient safety through regular physical checks, patient education, and the use of safety protocols (e.g., fall risk assessments).	AI-driven monitoring systems that use sensors to detect falls or environmental hazards, robotic assistants to help with patient mobility, and drones to deliver emergency supplies.
Communication	Direct nurse-patient interactions, telephone consultations, and written care plans.	Telehealth platforms for remote consultations, AI-powered virtual assistants for real-time communication, and chatbots for answering routine patient queries.
Breathing	Regular monitoring of respiratory rate and oxygen levels through physical assessment and basic monitoring tools.	AI-integrated monitoring devices that continuously track respiratory function, sending alerts for abnormalities, and nanobots that could potentially diagnose and treat respiratory conditions in real-time.
Eating and drinking	Manual feeding assistance, dietary planning, and fluid intake monitoring by nurses.	Automated feeding systems with AI to adjust diets based on real-time nutritional needs, smart utensils that monitor food intake, and remote dietary consultations via telehealth.

(Continued)

TABLE 7.2 (Continued)

Activities of Daily Living (ADLs) from RLT Model	Contemporary (Non-Digital) Application	Radical Digital/Technological Transformation
Elimination	Nurses assist with toileting needs, monitor urinary and bowel function, and provide incontinence care.	Smart toilets and urinary sensors that monitor output and detect abnormalities, AI-driven management systems for timely interventions, and robots to assist with toileting tasks.
Personal cleansing and dressing	Nurses provide assistance with bathing, grooming, and dressing, especially for patients with mobility challenges.	Robotic assistive devices that help with bathing and dressing, AI-enhanced wearables that track hygiene routines, and virtual reality (VR) training for patients to improve self-care skills.
Controlling body temperature	Regular temperature checks by nurses using thermometers, and manual adjustments to the environment (e.g., blankets, fans).	Smart wearables that continuously monitor body temperature and automatically adjust environmental controls (e.g., smart thermostats), and AI algorithms that predict and prevent hypothermia or hyperthermia.
Mobilising	Nurses assist patients with movement, transfers, and ambulation using physical strength or mobility aids.	Exoskeletons and robotic mobility aids that support patient movement, AI-driven rehabilitation platforms that guide and monitor mobility exercises, and drones for rapid transport of mobility aids.
Working and playing	Occupational therapy involving physical activities, games, and social interactions to promote mental and physical well-being.	Virtual reality (VR) environments that simulate work or play scenarios for therapeutic purposes, AI-driven platforms that recommend activities based on patient preferences and needs, and social robots for companionship and interactive games.
Expressing sexuality	Sensitive discussions facilitated by nurses, with support for sexual health and intimate relationships.	Telehealth consultations for sexual health, AI-driven apps providing personalised sexual health advice, and virtual reality (VR) to address sexual health issues in a safe, simulated environment.
Sleeping	Nurses monitor sleep patterns through observation, provide sleep hygiene education, and manage environmental factors.	AI-powered sleep monitors that track sleep cycles and suggest interventions, smart beds that adjust for optimal sleep, and telehealth platforms for sleep consultations.
Dying	End-of-life care provided by nurses, focusing on pain management, emotional support, and dignity.	AI-driven predictive tools that assess end-of-life needs, robotic palliative care assistants for routine tasks, and telehealth platforms for remote palliative care consultations and support.

the contemporary, largely non-digital applications of the RLT model with a radical vision for how these activities may be delivered using advanced technologies such as artificial intelligence, robotics, and telehealth.

Chapter summary

As we move further into the digital age, the future of nursing is increasingly intertwined with technology. This chapter has explored the profound impact that emerging technologies such as artificial intelligence, robotics, and telehealth are having on the nursing profession. These innovations promise to enhance the efficiency, accuracy, and scope of nursing care, yet they also present significant challenges, particularly regarding the preservation of compassionate care and the therapeutic relationship between nurse and patient. The transformation of nursing roles can be vividly illustrated via analysis using traditional models like the Roper, Logan, and Tierney framework but also indicates the need development of new models and philosophies that integrate digital tools while maintaining the core values of nursing. It is crucial that nurses remain at the forefront of this transformation, not only as practitioners but as leaders and innovators. By actively participating in the design, implementation, and regulation of healthcare technologies, nurses can ensure that these tools are used ethically and effectively, preserving the essence of nursing care while embracing the efficiencies that technology offers.

Nurse leaders must be courageous in questioning and reimagining the foundational concepts of nursing practice, such as compassionate care and the therapeutic relationship, in light of technological advancements. This involves advocating for robust education in technology and data science for nurses, ensuring that they are equipped to navigate and shape the digital landscape of healthcare. As we look towards the future, several critical questions arise: *What precisely must, if any, the roles of human nurses within healthcare systems be? How can we ensure that the integration of technology into nursing practice does not erode any essential human presence that is central to patient care? What new skills and competencies will nurses need to develop to thrive in a technology-driven healthcare environment? How can nurse leaders influence the development of technology to reflect the core values and purpose of the profession? And perhaps most importantly, what does it mean **to be a nurse** in a world where technology is increasingly taking over tasks traditionally performed by humans?*

In conclusion, the integration of technology into nursing is not an optional add-on but a necessary evolution that must be driven by those who understand the profession best: nurses themselves. By leading this charge, nurses can lay the foundation for a future where technology enhances, rather than diminishes, the quality of patient care. The questions posed are not just rhetorical, they are an invitation for all nurses to actively engage in shaping the future of their profession, ensuring that it remains vital, relevant, and patient-centred in the years to come.

References

Ayoub, M., Ballout, A. A., Zayek, R. A., & Ayoub, N. F. (2023). Mind + machine: ChatGPT as a basic clinical decisions support tool. *Cureus, 15*(8), e43690. https://doi.org/10.7759/cureus.43690

Bhatt, K., Pourmand, A., & Sikka, N. (2018). Targeted applications of unmanned aerial vehicles (drones) in telemedicine. *Telemedicine Journal and E-Health: The Official Journal of the American Telemedicine Association, 24*(11), 833–838.

Booth, R. G., Strudwick, G., McBride, S., O'Connor, S., & López, A. L. S. (2021). How the nursing profession should adapt for a digital future. *BMJ, 373*, n1190.

Brakmane, G., Khalifa, A., & Kattan, S. (2012). Nanobots in drug delivery. *Journal of Drug Delivery Science and Technology, 22*(6), 651–661.

Buchanan, C., Howitt, M. L., Wilson, R., Booth, R. G., Risling, T., & Bamford, M. (2020). Predicted influences of artificial intelligence on the domains of nursing: Scoping review. *JMIR Nursing, 3*(1), e23939.

Chakravarthy, K., Nagaraj, H., Darragh, A., & Kluger, M. (2018). The role of nanotechnology in pain management. *Pain Management, 8*(2), 113–126.

Conte, G., Arrigoni, C., Magon, A., Stievano, A., & Caruso, R. (2023). Embracing digital and technological solutions in nursing: A scoping review and conceptual framework. *International Journal of Medical Informatics, 177*, 105148.

Dobrina, R., Tenze, M., & Palese, A. (2014). An overview of hospice and palliative care nursing models and theories. *International Journal of Palliative Nursing, 20*(2), 75–81.

Earnshaw, V. A., Eaton, L. A., Kalichman, S. C., Brousseau, N. M., Hill, E. C., & Fox, A. B. (2020). COVID-19 conspiracy beliefs, health behaviors, and policy support. *Translational Behavioral Medicine*. https://doi.org/10.1093/tbm/ibaa090

Gharouifard, M., Zamanzadeh, V., Valizadeh, L., & Rahmani, A. (2022). Compassionate nursing care model: Results from a grounded theory study. *Nursing Ethics, 29*(3), 621–635.

Gibelli, F., Ricci, G., Sirignano, A., Turrina, S., & De Leo, D. (2021). The increasing centrality of robotic technology in the context of nursing care: Bioethical implications analyzed through a scoping review approach. *Journal of Healthcare Engineering, 2021*, 1478025. https://doi.org/10.1155/2021/1478025

Hants, L., Bail, K., & Paterson, C. (2023). Clinical decision-making and the nursing process in digital health systems: An integrated systematic review. *Journal of Clinical Nursing, 32*(19–20), 7010–7035.

Jafari, N., Lim, M., Hassani, A., Cordeiro, J., Kam, C., & Ho, K. (2022). Human-like tele-health robotics for older adults – A preliminary feasibility trial and vision. *Journal of Rehabilitation and Assistive Technologies Engineering, 9*, 20556683221140345.

Jain, Y., Lanjewar, R., & Shinde, R. K. (2024). Revolutionising breast surgery: A comprehensive review of robotic innovations in breast surgery and reconstruction. *Cureus, 16*(1), e52695.

Kangasniemi, M., Karki, S., Colley, N., & Voutilainen, A. (2019). The use of robots and other automated devices in nurses' work: An integrative review. *International Journal of Nursing Practice, 25*(4), e12739.

Kumar, S., Singh, H., Feder-Kubis, J., & Nguyen, D. D. (2023). Recent advances in nano-biosensors for sustainable healthcare applications: A systematic literature review. *Environmental Research, 238*, 117177.

Lee, D., Seong, M., Ju, H., & Park, M. (2024). Development of a nursing diagnosis/record generative AI system based on virtual patient data. *Studies in Health Technology and Informatics, 315*, 678–679.

Li, H., Zhu, G., Zhong, Y., Zhang, Z., Li, S., & Liu, J. (2024a). Applications of artificial intelligence in psychiatric nursing: A scope review. *Studies in Health Technology and Informatics, 315*, 74–80.

Li, Y., Wang, M., Wang, L., Cao, Y., Liu, Y., Zhao, Y., Yuan, R., Yang, M., Lu, S., Sun, Z., Zhou, F., Qian, Z., & Kang, H. (2024b). Advances in the application of AI robots in critical care: Scoping review. *Journal of Medical Internet Research, 26*, e54095.

Maalouf, N., Sidaoui, A., Elhajj, I. H., & Asmar, D. (2018). Robotics in nursing: A scoping review. *Journal of Nursing Scholarship: An Official Publication of Sigma Theta Tau International Honor Society of Nursing, 50*(6), 590–600.

McAllister, M., Dunn, G., Payne, K., Davies, L., Todd, C., & MacLeod, R. (2012). Empowerment: Qualitative underpinning of a new patient-reported outcome for personal recovery in psychosis. *BMC Psychiatry, 12*(1), 15.

Miczo, N. (2004). Stressors and social support perceptions predict illness attitudes and care-seeking intentions: Re-examining the sick role. *Health Communication, 16*(3), 347–361.

Mirhaghi, A., Sharafi, S., Bazzi, A., & Hasanzadeh, F. (2017). Therapeutic relationship: Is it still the heart of nursing? *Nursing Reports, 7*(1), 6129.

Moazemi, S., Vahdati, S., Li, J., Kalkhoff, S., Castano, L. J. V., Dewitz, B., Bibo, R., Sabouniaghdam, P., Tootooni, M. S., Bundschuh, R. A., Lichtenberg, A., Aubin, H., & Schmid, F. (2023). Artificial intelligence for clinical decision support for monitoring patients in cardiovascular ICUs: A systematic review. *Frontiers in Medicine, 10*, 1109411.

Mogueo, A., & Defo, B. K. (2022). Patients' and family caregivers' experiences and perceptions about factors hampering or facilitating patient empowerment for self-management of hypertension and diabetes in Cameroon. *BMC Health Services Research, 22*(1), 1381. https://doi.org/10.1186/s12913-022-08750-4

O'Connor, S., Cave, L., & Philips, N. (2024). Informing nursing policy: An exploration of digital health research by nurses in England. *International Journal of Medical Informatics, 185*, 105381.

O'Connor, S., Yan, Y., Thilo, F. J. S., Felzmann, H., Dowding, D., & Lee, J. J. (2023). Artificial intelligence in nursing and midwifery: A systematic review. *Journal of Clinical Nursing, 32*(13–14), 2951–2968.

Olawade, D. B., Wada, O. J., David-Olawade, A. C., Kunonga, E., Abaire, O., & Ling, J. (2023). Using artificial intelligence to improve public health: A narrative review. *Frontiers in Public Health, 11*, 1196397.

Orlando, I. J. (1961). *The dynamic nurse-patient relationship: Function, process, and principles.* New York: G.P. Putnam's Sons.

Papadopoulos, I., & Koulouglioti, C. (2018). The influence of culture on attitudes towards humanoid and animal-like robots: An integrative review. *Journal of Nursing Scholarship: An Official Publication of Sigma Theta Tau International Honor Society of Nursing, 50*(6), 653–665.

Ronquillo, C. E., Peltonen, L., Pruinelli, L., Chu, C. H., Bakken, S., Beduschi, A., Cato, K., Hardiker, N., Junger, A., Michalowski, M., Nyrup, R., Rahimi, S., Reed, D. N., Salakoski, T., Salanterä, S., Walton, N., Weber, P., Wiegand, T., & Topaz, M. (2021). Artificial intelligence in nursing: Priorities and opportunities from an international invitational think-tank of the Nursing and Artificial Intelligence Leadership Collaborative. *Journal of Advanced Nursing, 77*(9), 3707–3717.

Reddy, S. (2024). Generative AI in healthcare: An implementation science informed translational path on application, integration, and governance. *Implementation Science, 19*(1), 27.

Reddy, V., Nafees, A., & Raman, S. (2023). Recent advances in artificial intelligence applications for supportive and palliative care in cancer patients. *Current Opinion in Supportive and Palliative Care, 17*(2), 125–134.

Roper, N., Logan, W. W., & Tierney, A. J. (2000). *The Roper-Logan-Tierney model of nursing: Based on activities of living.* Edinburgh: Churchill Livingstone.

Rony, M. K. K., Parvin, M. R., & Ferdousi, S. (2024). Advancing nursing practice with artificial intelligence: Enhancing preparedness for the future. *Nursing Open, 11*(1). https://doi.org/10.1002/nop2.2070

Russo, G., Moretta Tartaglione, A., & Cavacece, Y. (2019). Empowering patients to co-create a sustainable healthcare value. *Sustainability, 11*(5), 1315. https://doi.org/10.3390/su11051315

Schmidt, B. J., & McArthur, E. C. (2018). Professional nursing values: A concept analysis. *Nursing Forum, 53*(1), 69–75.

Servaty, R., Kersten, A., Brukamp, K., Möhler, R., & Mueller, M. (2020). Implementation of robotic devices in nursing care. Barriers and facilitators: An integrative review. *BMJ Open, 10*(9), e038650.

Sharman, J. (2023). Recognising and addressing health misinformation in nursing practice. *Primary Health Care, 4*, 24–29.

Shaw, R. J. (2023). Access to technology and digital literacy as determinants of health and health care. *Creative Nursing, 29*(3), 258–263.

Strudwick, G., & Risling, T. (2024). Beyond the hype: It's time for nursing to take a close look at artificial intelligence. *Canadian Nurse.* ePub ahead of print. Retrieved from https://www.ams-inc.on.ca/wp-content/uploads/2020/02/Nursing-and-Compassionate-Care.pdf

Strudwick, G., Wiljer, D., & Inglis, F. (2020). *Nursing and compassionate care in a technological world: A discussion paper.* Toronto: AMS Healthcare.

Tischendorf, T., Heitmann-Möller, A., Ruppert, S., Marchwacka, M., Schaffrin, S., Schaal, T., & Hasseler, M. (2024). Sustainable integration of digitalisation in nursing education—An international scoping review. *Frontiers in Health Services, 4*, 1344021.

World Health Organization. (2020). *State of the world's nursing 2020: Investing in education, jobs, and leadership.* Geneva: World Health Organization. Retrieved from https://iris.who.int/bitstream/handle/10665/331677/9789240003279-eng.pdf?sequence=1

Wynn, M., Garwood-Cross, L., Vasilica, C., & Davis, D. (2023). Digital nursing practice theory: A scoping review and thematic analysis. *Journal of Advanced Nursing, 79*(11), 4137–4150.

Zafrani, O., & Nimrod, G. (2019). Towards a holistic approach to studying human-robot interaction in later life. *The Gerontologist, 59*(1), e26–e36.

INDEX

Note: **Bold** page numbers refer to tables and *italic* page numbers refer to figures.

Printed in the United States
by Baker & Taylor Publisher Services